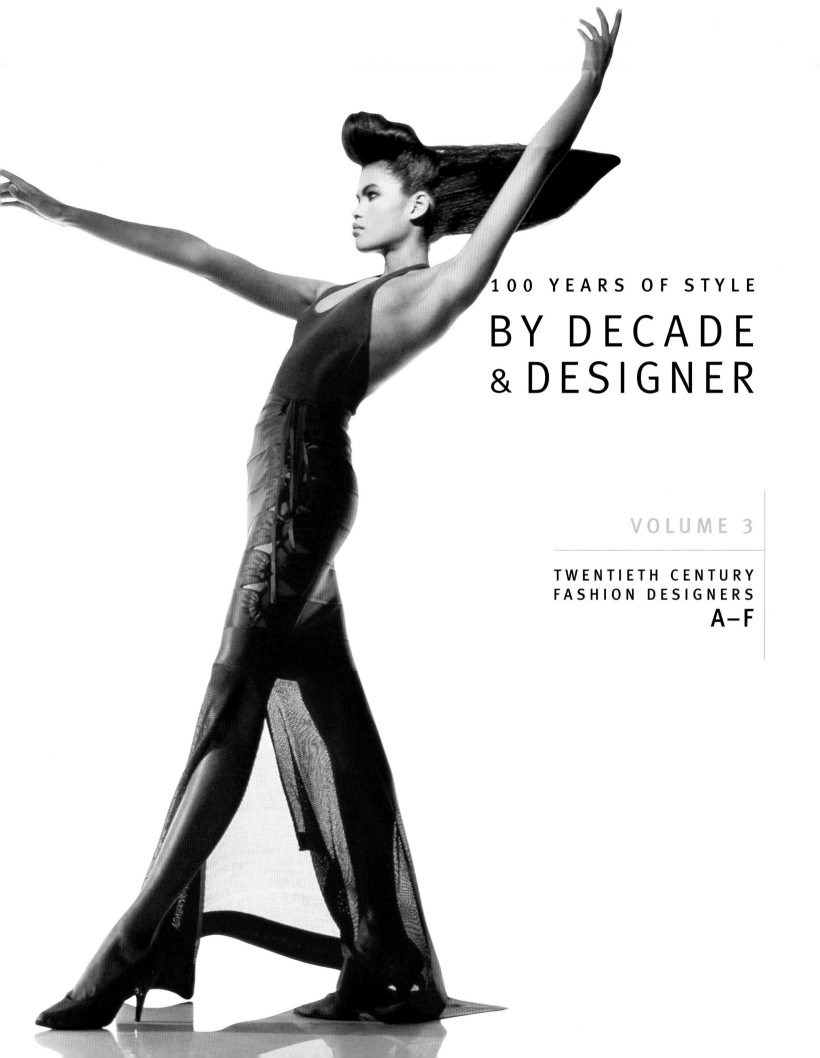

100 YEARS OF STYLE

BY DECADE
& DESIGNER

VOLUME 3

TWENTIETH CENTURY
FASHION DESIGNERS
A–F

First printing

1 3 5 7 9 8 6 4 2

The Chelsea House World Wide Web address is
http://www.chelseahouse.com

Library of Congress Cataloging-in-Publication Data applied for

ISBN 0 7910 6194 9 Fashion Designers A–F (this edition)

0 7910 6192 2 Fashions 1900–1949

0 7910 6193 0 Fashions 1950–1999

0 7910 6195 7 Fashion Designers G–M

0 7910 6196 5 Fashion Designers N–Z

0 7910 6191 4 (set)

Produced by Carlton Books
20 Mortimer Street
London W1N 7RD

Text and Design copyright © Carlton Books Limited 1999/2000

Photographs copyright © 1999 Condé Nast Publications Limited

Previous page: 'Shapeliness Nouveau' from Azzedine Alaïa, 1986. Tomato-red acetate knit halter and corset-strapped skirt 'tied tight as tight down one side'.

Opposite: Comme des Garçons' angular jacket of 1986 'with maverick swagged peplum', in Venetian striped polyester satin.

Overleaf: Kingsize djellaba supercover by John Bates, in black wool crepe; striped, bound, panelled in flowers of embroidered ultraviolet silk, 1972.

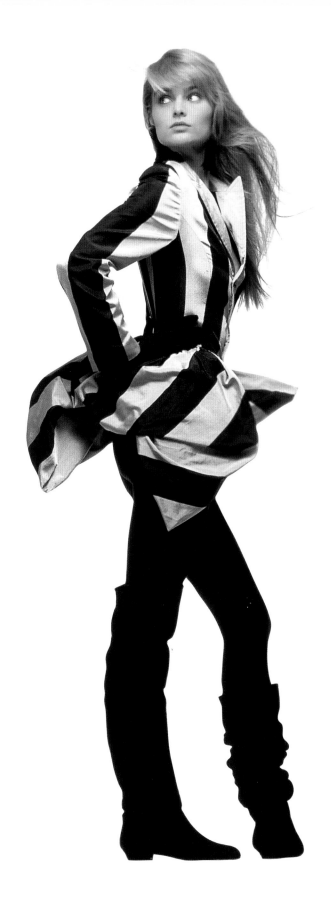

100 YEARS OF STYLE
BY DECADE
& DESIGNER

Linda Watson

VOLUME 3

TWENTIETH CENTURY
FASHION DESIGNERS
A–F

Chelsea House Publishers

PHILADELPHIA

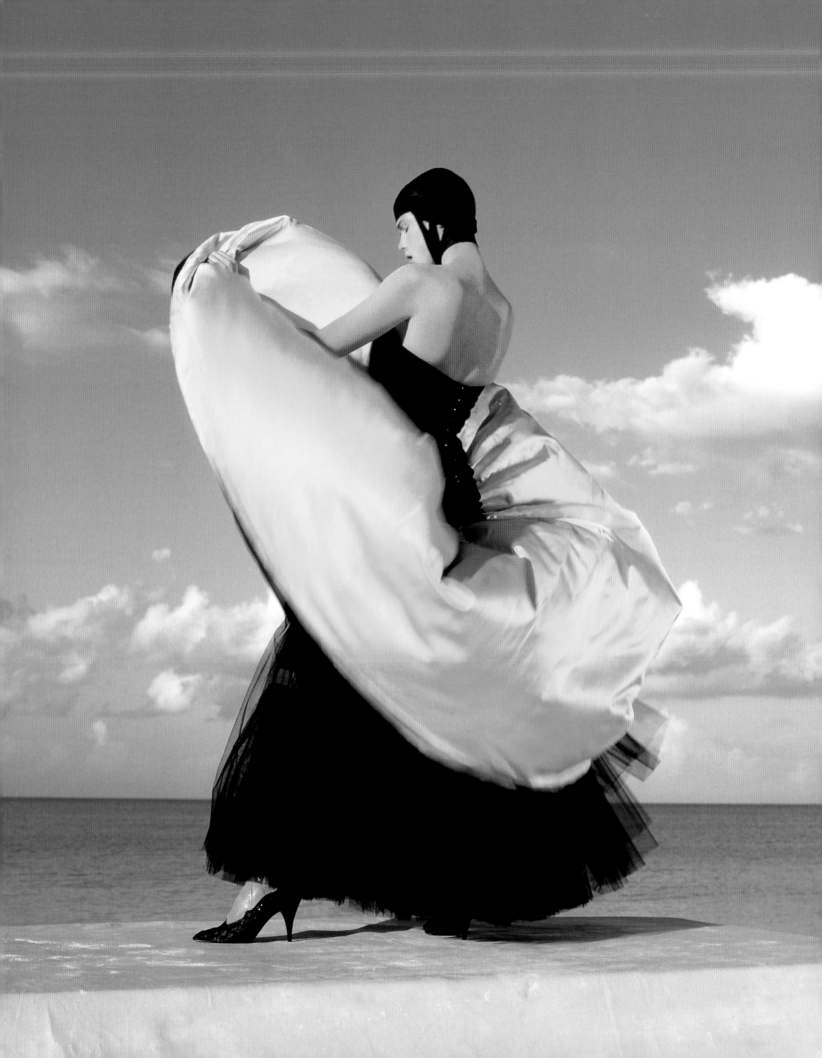

contents

ADOLFO

BORN: CARDENAS, CUBA, 1933

'Since Nancy Reagan, one of Adolfo's biggest fans, has become first lady, the crush to get a front-row seat became an upmanship scene,' reported American *Vogue* magazine in 1981. Designer to New York's socially significant, Adolfo's first client was Gloria Vanderbilt and his most famous was Nancy Reagan, for whom he made a red wool inauguration coat and matching braided toque.

When Adolfo closed his New York salon in April 1993, it signalled the end of an era, which began in 1948 when Adolfo F Sardina arrived in New York from Cuba. Like Halston, Adolfo initially trained as a milliner, before working first at Bergdorf Goodman and then at Emme. In 1967 he established his own ready-to-wear business. The Adolfo look was never experimental, rather a quiet classic style – with shades of Chanel – which enabled the wearer to glide effortlessly through social situations.

ADRIAN, Gilbert

BORN: NAUGATUCK, CONNECTICUT, USA, 1903
DIED: LOS ANGELES, CALIFORNIA, USA, 1959

'Twelve hundred costumes, five thousand wigs and fripperies for two poodles were Adrian's pre-occupation during the filming of *Marie Antionette*,' noted *Vogue* in 1938. The most prolific costume designer of Hollywood's heyday, Gilbert Adrian's square 'coathanger' shoulders and elongated silhouette captured the audiences and knocked Paris off kilter. Adrian designed for every Hollywood beauty, including Jean Harlow in *Dinner at Eight* (1933), Joan Crawford in *Letty Lyndon* (1932) and Katharine Hepburn in *The Philadelphia Story* (1940). His first film costumes were for Rudolph Valentino in *The Eagle* in 1925.

Adrian – born Adrian Adolph Greenburg – had creativity in his genes: his father ran a millinery business, his mother was an artist, his uncle a theatrical designer. In 1921 he enrolled at Parson's School of Design in New York to study fashion and was transferred to Paris, where he met Irving Berlin.

He returned to New York, designing for Berlin's *Music Box Reviews*, before moving to Paramount to work with the film producer and director Cecil B de Mille.

In 1941 he formed Adrian Limited, a ready-to-wear business based in Beverly Hills, and showed his first collection the following year. He launched two complementary fragrances, Saint and Sinner, in 1946 and opened a boutique in New York in 1948. After suffering a heart attack, he retired with his wife, actress Janet Gaynor, to recuperate in Brazil. In 1959 Adrian died, having returned to his first love, designing costumes for the Lerner and Loewe production, *Camelot*.

AGNÈS B

BORN: VERSAILLES, FRANCE, 1943

Eclectic, young and with the simplicity of a school uniform, the Agnès B label has branches in London, Tokyo, Los Angeles and Amsterdam. Her first customer was actress Dominique Sandra.

In the mid-1970s, having worked as a fashion editor and assistant to designer Dorothée Bis, Agnès B designed her own collection and opened a boutique in 1976. Agnès B also designs specifically for teenagers and children, and produced a maternity collection: fitting for a woman who at 43 had four children and one grandchild. 'I always make things I would wear,' she told *Vogue* in 1986. 'I love white, I love black, and I love finding new colours. I think people like my clothes because they can be neutral.'

AGNÈS, Madame

BORN: FRANCE, LATE 1800S
(ACTIVE: 1910–40)

Agnès hats, named after their maker, appeared regularly in *Vogue* in the 1920s and 1930s. She could turn her hand to the occasional incredible concoction, but mostly Madame Agnès made chic cloches, swirling felts and variations on a beret that had been popularized by Marlene Dietrich. During the 1920s millinery was a fine art which became an occupation of the chic, and Madame Agnès, photographed by *Vogue* in 1925 wearing a futurist dress and angular earrings – influenced by the Cubists – was a prime example.

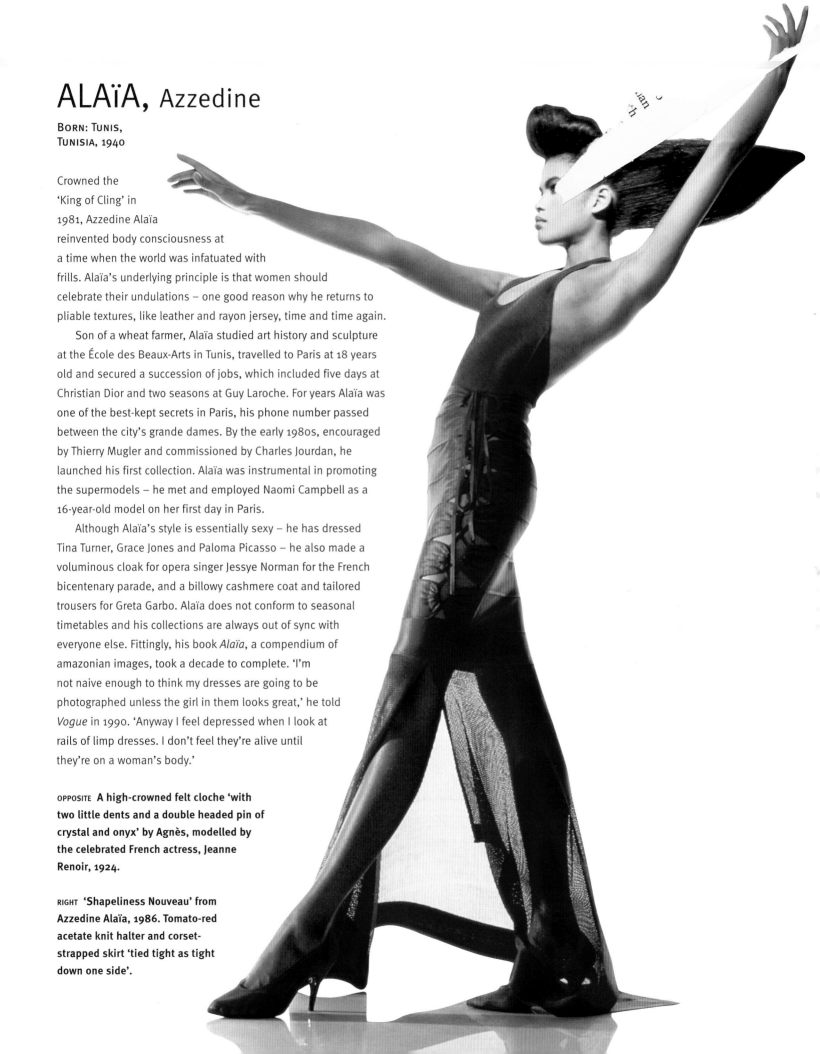

ALAïA, Azzedine

BORN: TUNIS,
TUNISIA, 1940

Crowned the
'King of Cling' in
1981, Azzedine Alaïa
reinvented body consciousness at
a time when the world was infatuated with
frills. Alaïa's underlying principle is that women should
celebrate their undulations – one good reason why he returns to
pliable textures, like leather and rayon jersey, time and time again.

Son of a wheat farmer, Alaïa studied art history and sculpture
at the École des Beaux-Arts in Tunis, travelled to Paris at 18 years
old and secured a succession of jobs, which included five days at
Christian Dior and two seasons at Guy Laroche. For years Alaïa was
one of the best-kept secrets in Paris, his phone number passed
between the city's grande dames. By the early 1980s, encouraged
by Thierry Mugler and commissioned by Charles Jourdan, he
launched his first collection. Alaïa was instrumental in promoting
the supermodels – he met and employed Naomi Campbell as a
16-year-old model on her first day in Paris.

Although Alaïa's style is essentially sexy – he has dressed
Tina Turner, Grace Jones and Paloma Picasso – he also made a
voluminous cloak for opera singer Jessye Norman for the French
bicentenary parade, and a billowy cashmere coat and tailored
trousers for Greta Garbo. Alaïa does not conform to seasonal
timetables and his collections are always out of sync with
everyone else. Fittingly, his book *Alaïa*, a compendium of
amazonian images, took a decade to complete. 'I'm
not naive enough to think my dresses are going to be
photographed unless the girl in them looks great,' he told
Vogue in 1990. 'Anyway I feel depressed when I look at
rails of limp dresses. I don't feel they're alive until
they're on a woman's body.'

OPPOSITE **A high-crowned felt cloche 'with
two little dents and a double headed pin of
crystal and onyx' by Agnès, modelled by
the celebrated French actress, Jeanne
Renoir, 1924.**

RIGHT **'Shapeliness Nouveau' from
Azzedine Alaïa, 1986. Tomato-red
acetate knit halter and corset-
strapped skirt 'tied tight as tight
down one side'.**

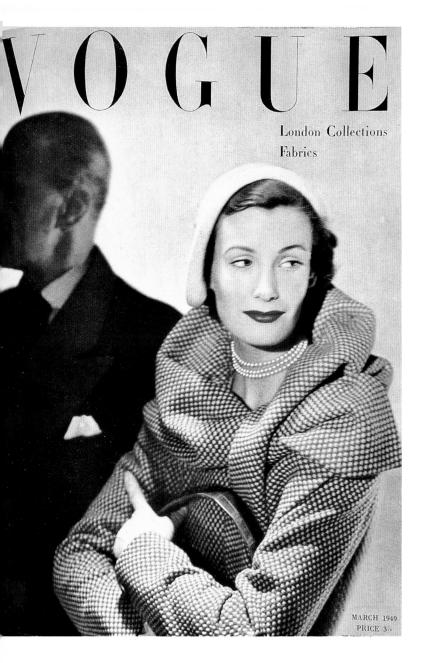

VOGUE

London Collections
Fabrics

MARCH 1949
PRICE 3/-

LEFT **Hardy Amies' first** *Vogue*
cover, March 1949, photographed
by Norman Parkinson, shows
an Amies shawl-collared jacket
with ubiquitous pearls and
Agmar cloche.

OPPOSITE **Giorgio Armani's**
sequinned 'sunbeaded'
sarong dress with shoestring
shoulder straps, worn by
supermodel Claudia
Schiffer in 1991.

AMIES, Sir Hardy

BORN: LONDON, ENGLAND, 1909

England's most distinguished designer has become something
of an *enfant terrible* in his old age, frequently consulted by style
pundits for his outspoken opinions on everything from modern
manners to the minutiae of old-fashioned roses (his favourite is
a subtly striped variety called *Rosa* 'Mundi').

Hardy Amies was educated at Brentwood. His father was a
London County Council surveyor, his mother a *vendeuse* at a court
dressmaker called Miss Gray Limited. In 1934 he became head
designer at Lachasse, taking over from Digby Morton. During the

Second World War, Amies, who was fluent in French and German,
joined the Intelligence Corps, working for the Special Operations
Executive as head of the Belgium section, organizing the dropping
of Resistance workers during the occupation. In 1945 he opened
his house at 14 Savile Row, London, a property formerly owned by
restoration playwright, Richard Brinsley Sheridan. He presented his
own-name collection the following year. Hardy Amies has been the
Queen's dressmaker since 1950, when Princess Elizabeth, as she
was then, made her first royal tour of Canada. He has made clothes
for every royal tour since, his *pièce de résistance* being the pink
dress the Queen wore in Jubilee year.

Described by *Vogue* in 1960 as 'a brisk, dynamic man with
a finger in innumerable pies', Hardy Amies has always been
a vigorous promoter of his own business. In the early 1960s he
frequently travelled to America and Australia on promotional
tours. By 1964 he was head of a successful business, which
included couture, a boutique and a ready-to-wear collection,
and had a turnover of £15 million in menswear and £750,000
in womenswear. He owns a flat in London's Kensington and
a converted Victorian school in Gloucestershire.

Amies has witnessed a very significant fashion revolution of
the twentieth century and has made a valuable contribution to
British fashion: first to the Government's wartime utility scheme,
which made Britain count on the world stage, and secondly,
incisively predicting the onset of the New Look. The house is now
run by design director Jon Moore, and menswear by Ian Garlant;
but, at 90 years of age, Sir Hardy still works a three-day week.

Hardy Amies was awarded a CVO in 1977 and in 1989
a KCVO – a non-political knighthood awarded only to those
who work closely with the Queen. He has published two
autobiographies, *Just So Far*, in 1954, and *Still Here*, 30 years
later. A decade after that he wrote *The Englishman's Suit* –
a wry look at sartorial propriety. Speaking about style to *Vogue*
in 1984 he said, 'The greatest enemy of style is gentility because
style is honesty.' At his spring/summer 1999 couture show,
Sir Hardy, immaculately dressed and sitting at the back of the
salon, instructed the audience to savour the moment. 'Why
don't you clap?' he said loudly while the models were mid-
twirl, 'It's a *marvellous* outfit.'

ARMANI, Giorgio

BORN: PIACENZA, ITALY, 1934

'In Italy, fashion is logical, rational and wearable,' observed Giorgio Armani in 1986. 'I do not allow myself the luxury of waiting for inspiration. The birth of a new collection is a drama, of course. But in the end I sit down alone at a sheet of white paper, and design.' Architect of the soft shoulder and fluid suit, Giorgio Armani is the undisputed king of Italian tailoring, revered by his contemporaries and customers alike.

Having studied medicine at the University of Bologna, Armani left in 1953 to serve in the Italian army. In 1954 he was employed as a window-display designer and stylist, and eventually became menswear buyer for La Rinascente department store chain. He designed menswear for Nino Cerruti from 1960–70, followed by five years of freelance work, culminating in the launch of his own menswear collection, instigated by his close friend and business partner Sergio Galeotti in 1975.

Armani spent almost 20 years analysing fashion from different angles – and it shows. He sees clothes in the round and the fashion industry as a complete entity, its quiet evolution rather than earth-moving revolution. He isn't into trickery. He sells. He delivers. No wonder Armani is the biggest-selling European designer in the USA. Myths and legends surround the designer with his white hair, permanent tan and calm veneer, but the picture

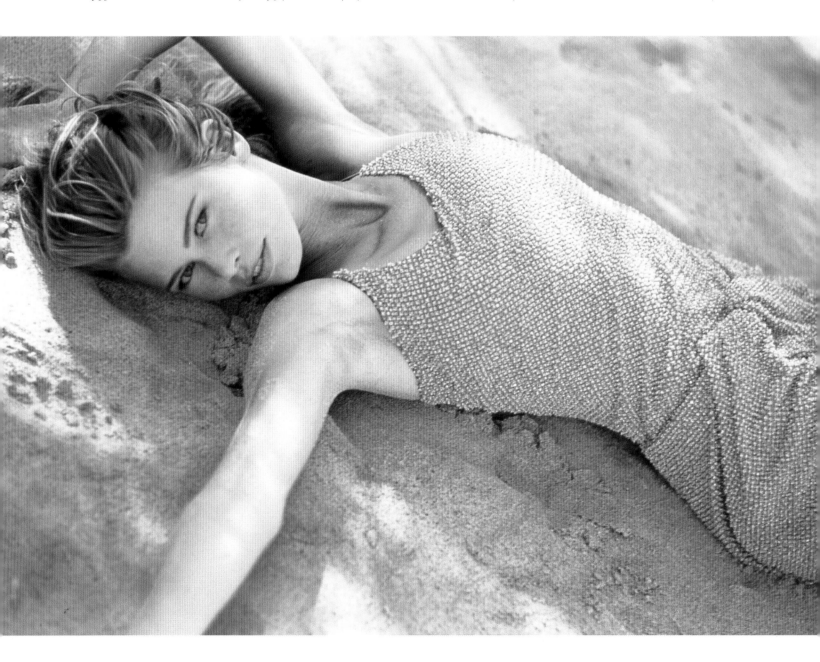

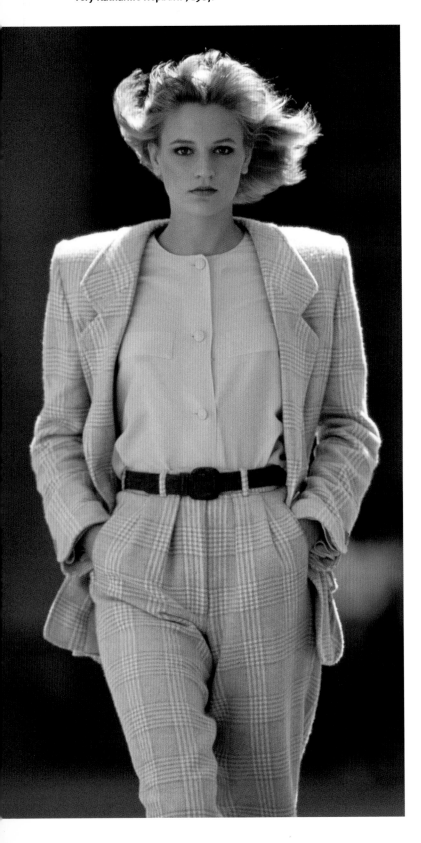

emerges of a perfectionist who dictates the precise distance between hangers, allows his cats to eat from starched white napkins, and only handles credit cards, never cash. His staff say he resembles Rodin's *Thinker* while designing.

During the designer decade, Armani was the symbol of success among the stockbrokers and financial whiz kids around the world – a quiet, assured label which spoke a thousand words about salary levels and business hierarchy. The recipient of numerous awards, Armani's accolades include the Grand Ufficiale dell'Ordine al Merito della Republica – the highest government award – and a doctorate from the Royal College of Art. His doctorate for design excellence put him on a par with architect Sir Norman Foster and David Lynch, director of *Twin Peaks* (1989).

Armani always has a strong presence at the Oscars and has dressed the A-list of screen stars including Jodie Foster, Anjelica Huston, Michelle Pfeiffer and Robert de Niro. He made clothes for *The Untouchables* (1987) and *American Gigolo* (1980). The director Martin Scorsese made a 26-minute documentary film about Armani's collection, called *Made in Milan*, which was launched at the Venice film festival in September 1990. Armani now has a Los Angeles representative to coordinate celebrity clients but in 1987 he protested, 'Please don't call me a celebrity designer. I like designing for people who work, so that includes actors and actresses, but as people who work, not as stars.'

ASHLEY, Laura

BORN: MERTHYR TYDFIL, WALES, 1925
DIED: COVENTRY, ENGLAND, 1985

Advocate of the piecrust frill and full-blown ballgown, Laura Ashley began her business by silk-screen printing textiles on her kitchen table. Together with her husband, Bernard, Ashley started selling scarves to John Lewis. Laura Ashley Limited was established in 1968 when the couple opened their first outlet in Pelham Street, Kensington. The design ethos – puffed sleeves, smocks and voluminous dresses with patch pockets – were available in a variety of pretty cotton prints, including stripes, spots and floral sprigs. At its height – during the 1960s, 1970s and 1980s – there were Laura Ashley shops in Paris, Geneva, New York and San Francisco. By the 1980s Laura Ashley sold lawn fabrics, printed cottons and linens. In 1977 she won the Queen's Award for Export Achievement. Laura Ashley turned down an OBE because her husband wasn't offered one too, but Buckingham Palace made amends in 1987 and gave him a knighthood. As a consequence of boardroom shuffles and shifting fashion tastes, the company's philosophy started to waver after Laura Ashley's death. Today, Laura Ashley remains a strong presence on the high street, but the designs have a twist on the English rose and elegant eveningwear rubs shoulders with anonymous tunics, but the traditional ethos is still apparent – with cotton summer dresses evoking thoughts of garden parties, and cable-knit sweaters prompting memories of long weekends spent in the country.

AUGUSTABERNARD

FOUNDED BY AUGUSTA BERNARD IN 1919

'The new silhouette slides in like a fish', observed *Vogue* in its 'Turning Points towards a New Mode' in 1933. 'Augustabernard was the magician who first called it to life. This silhouette is vertical, but well formed; it makes a woman look extremely tall, but at the same time rounded. No extreme bulk, but the natural, normal curves of the figure.'

Augustabernard opened in 1919 – its founder linking her Christian and surname together to form the name. She became famous for her bias cutting, slim silhouettes and ability to excel in flattery. Her designs were spare and intricate in construction; like Madeleine Vionnet, Augustabernard was a technical wizard. Unfortunately, during the depression of the 1930s, her clients started to tighten their belts and Augustabernard, sadly, slid out of business as a result.

BAKST, Léon

BORN: ST PETERSBURG, RUSSIA, 1866
DIED: PARIS, FRANCE, 1924

A fine artist turned costume designer, Léon Bakst was best known for his work with the Ballets Russes, where his exotic use of colour and extraordinary patterns had a profound influence on fashion. His costume designs – drawn mainly on Greek and Egyptian lines – often combined inverted triangles and vertical lines. Bakst gave lectures on the aesthetic principles of dress during the 1920s. He analysed the slim silhouette for *Vogue*, showing how the positioning of graphic pattern could destroy or enhance a silhouette, and stressed the importance of having a beautiful body. 'Like a magnificent dog or horse – forgive, Mesdames, this comparison since it is in your praise – the woman who possesses beautiful articulation is a woman of race: sick or well, she always bears the mark of physical perfection.'

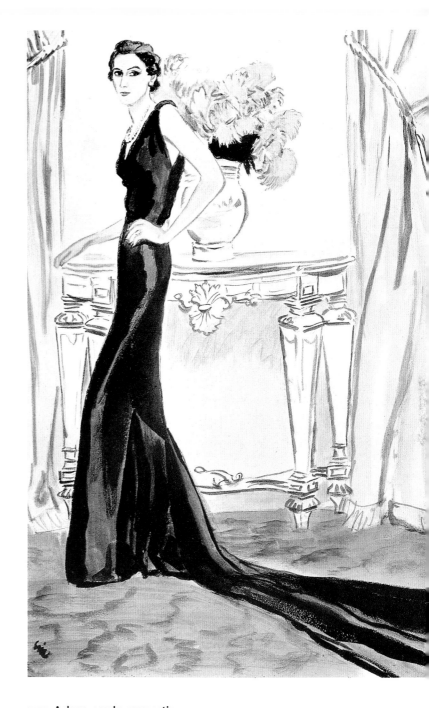

ABOVE **A deep, smoke-grey satin sheath from Augustabernard for 'modern sirens who lend such enchantement to the drawing-room', 1934.**

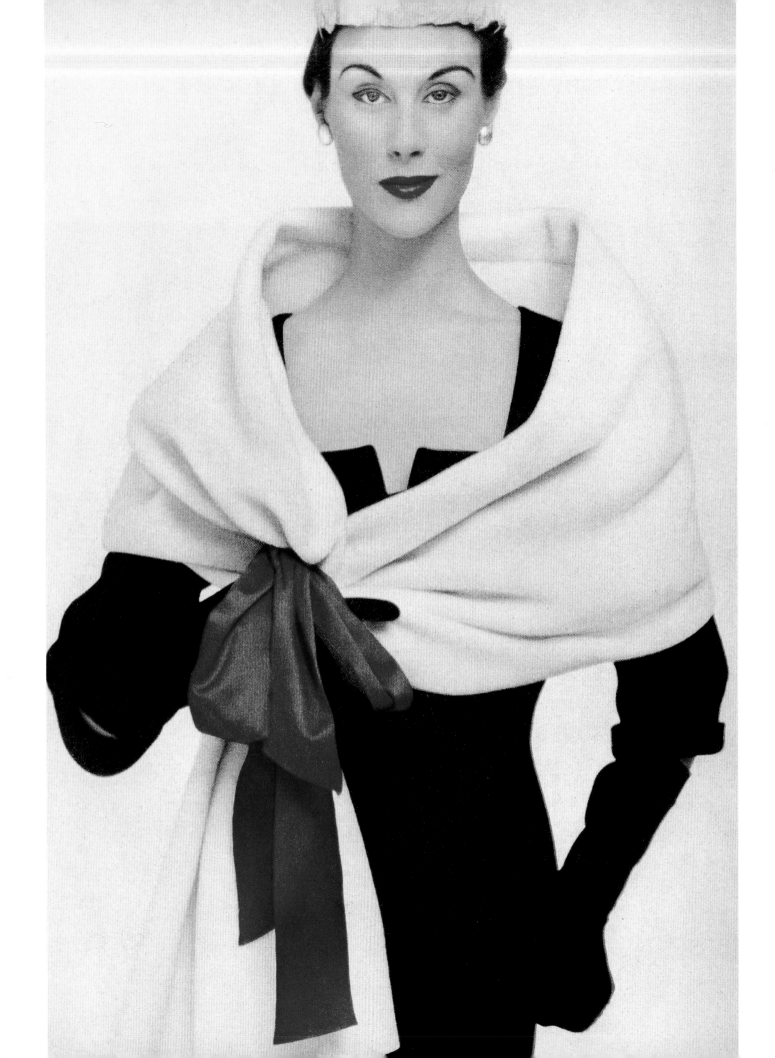

BALENCIAGA, Cristobal

BORN: GUETARIA, SPAIN, 1895

DIED: JAVEA, SPAIN, 1972

In *Vogue*, 1962: 'There is one brief, pithy Spanish word, *cursi*, that Balenciaga uses to describe what he hates most in fashion: vulgarity and bad taste. Of these he has never, ever, been guilty.' Cristobal Balenciaga is the undisputed designer's designer. Revered and admired by couturiers past and present, including a coterie of all-time greats: Madeleine Vionnet, Hubert de Givenchy, Christian Dior and Coco Chanel. André Courrèges and Emanuel Ungaro were lucky enough to have worked with him on a one-to-one basis. Givenchy, for whom Balenciaga was a mentor, described him to *Vogue* in 1991 as 'Gracious, elegant, religious, simple, talented.'

Balenciaga's colour palette was, like his clothes, very carefully edited. 'His colours are of Spain', commented *Vogue* in 1962, 'deep, thick black, accented with white; brilliant reds; turquoise; yellow; warm, cinnamon browns; and whether he knows it or not, Goya is always looking over his shoulder.' The immaculate quality of his collections prompted *Vogue* to observe that what Balenciaga designed in 1938 would always transcend time. 'He has a complete and utter disregard for public opinion, caring not a fig whether Press or customers like his collection, and because he follows no ideas or trends but his own, everyone follows him.'

Balenciaga was the son of a fisherman and seamstress. One of his mother's clients, the Marquesa de Casa Torres, apprenticed him to a tailor at 13 years old. At 24 he opened his own house, dressing ladies of the court of Alphonse XIII. Balenciaga went bankrupt in 1931, reopened in Madrid and Barcelona, and travelled to Paris, via London, six years later. In the latter part of his career, Balenciaga was asked to lend his name to an American tie line. He felt licensing was a form of prostitution. Givenchy recalled, 'He was indeed of another era. When commissioned to design Air France uniforms he wanted to personally do the fittings for 3,000 stewardesses.'

Unlike Dior, who made a statement which changed the course of twentieth-century fashion, Balenciaga created the most enduring examples of perfection. In 1962 *Vogue* observed that Balenciaga was 'an implicit believer in the golden rule of fashion – that the essence of chic is elimination. It follows that he has the most elegant clientele in the world.' Six years later – a year before man landed on the moon – Balenciaga closed the doors to his business, claiming there was no one left for him to dress. When customers asked where they should go, 73-year-old Balenciaga pointed them in the direction of Givenchy, whose salon was situated across the street.

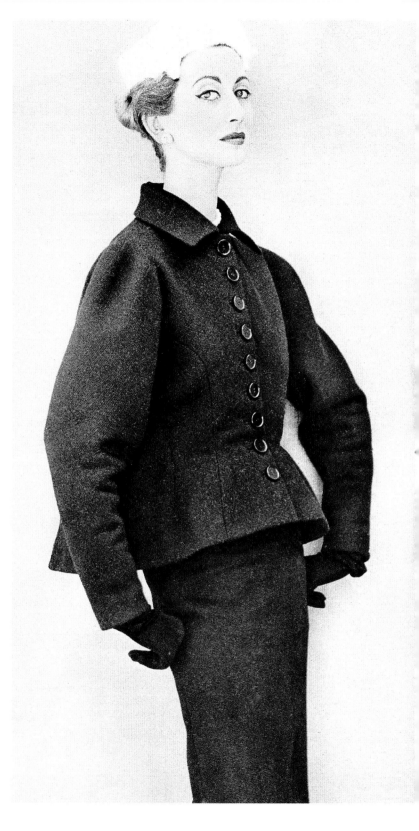

OPPOSITE **The 'revolutionary late-day variation on a suit-plus-stole theme', 1952 – a black suit, white stole and cyclamen ribbon.**

ABOVE **Balenciaga's structured suit of immaculate proportions: 'fitted front, loose back line' in black wool ottoman, September 1951.**

BALMAIN, Pierre

BORN: ST-JEAN-DE-MAURIENNE, FRANCE, 1914

DIED: PARIS, FRANCE, 1982

A mover rather than a shaker, Pierre Balmain launched his career by working with three of fashion's greats before branching out on his own. He began freelance drawing for Robert Piguet and then spent five years with Edward Molyneux before moving on to Lucien Lelong, where he sketched alongside a young designer called Christian Dior. Balmain's own Parisian house opened on 12 October 1945. His *pièce de résistance* was an embroidered white brocade dinner dress worth 120,000 francs.

Although Balmain's grandfather had owned a drapery business, financial difficulties prompted his mother to suggest that Pierre become a naval surgeon. He ignored her advice and instead, wrote to Piguet, Lelong, Jeanne Lanvin and Molyneux. The latter gave Balmain his first job. On his own, Balmain's clients included the Duchess of Windsor, the Duchess of Kent, Sophia Loren and the Queen of Siam.

Since his death in 1982, many designers have taken over the Balmain mantle: first Erik Mortensen, then Alistair Blair. In November 1992 Hervé Pierre was replaced by Oscar de la Renta. In his biography, *My Years and Seasons* published in 1964, Balmain reflected, 'Business turnover may grow, personnel change, publicity [become] more blatant, but a couture house seldom escapes from the category in which it is initially placed. I was lucky that my first show earned me a high rating.'

BANTON, Travis

BORN: WACO, TEXAS, USA, 1894

DIED: LOS ANGELES, CALIFORNIA, USA, 1958

Travis Banton was considered – along with Gilbert Adrian – one of the most important figures in Hollywood. Having attended the New York School of Fine and Applied Arts, he worked for Lucile Duff Gordon, who was then one of the most famous couturiers in the world. Banton's big break came in 1924, when he was commissioned to design the costumes for Leatrice Joy and the cast of *A Dressmaker in Paris*.

During his time as chief designer at Paramount, from 1927–38, Banton created costumes for Tallulah Bankhead, Marlene Dietrich, and Claudette Colbert's 1935 appearance in *Cleopatra*. His trademark was bias cutting and body consciousness. When his contract expired with Paramount, he switched to Twentieth-Century Fox, then Universal Studios.

BATES, John

BORN: DINNINGTON, ENGLAND, 1935

'I admire the way Americans care, but it shows a little and it shouldn't,' said John Bates in *Vogue*'s 'Designer Series' in 1976, 'they're best when they're wearing the least make-up and their hair shines like they invented shampoo.'

One of the brightest stars of British fashion during the 1970s, Bates had a French training at Herbert Sidon of Sloane Street in London; he then moved to Jean Varon in 1958 and formed his own label in 1972. Bates had a meticulous attention to detail, piecing together the complete look from millinery to custom-made stockings. He made his name by dressing Diana Rigg for *The Avengers* television series; her first outfit – a fight-scene suit with a black stripe across the bustline – was commissioned and made within three days.

Bates's business went bankrupt in 1980 and, faced with an uncertain future in the rag trade, otherwise known as the 'Calcutta run, which you do if you want to feel instantly depressed', he moved to Wales in 1989, where he lives in a cottage with views over the estuary, designing for larger ladies and perfecting his life-drawing technique.

LEFT **Balmain's Tibetan jacket, from his *Jolie Madame* collection of 1957, with sweeping sleeves and inner cuffs of leopardskin 'to match the helmet hat'.**

OPPOSITE **Kingsize djellaba super-cover by John Bates, in black wool crepe; striped, bound, panelled in flowers of embroidered ultraviolet silk, 1976.**

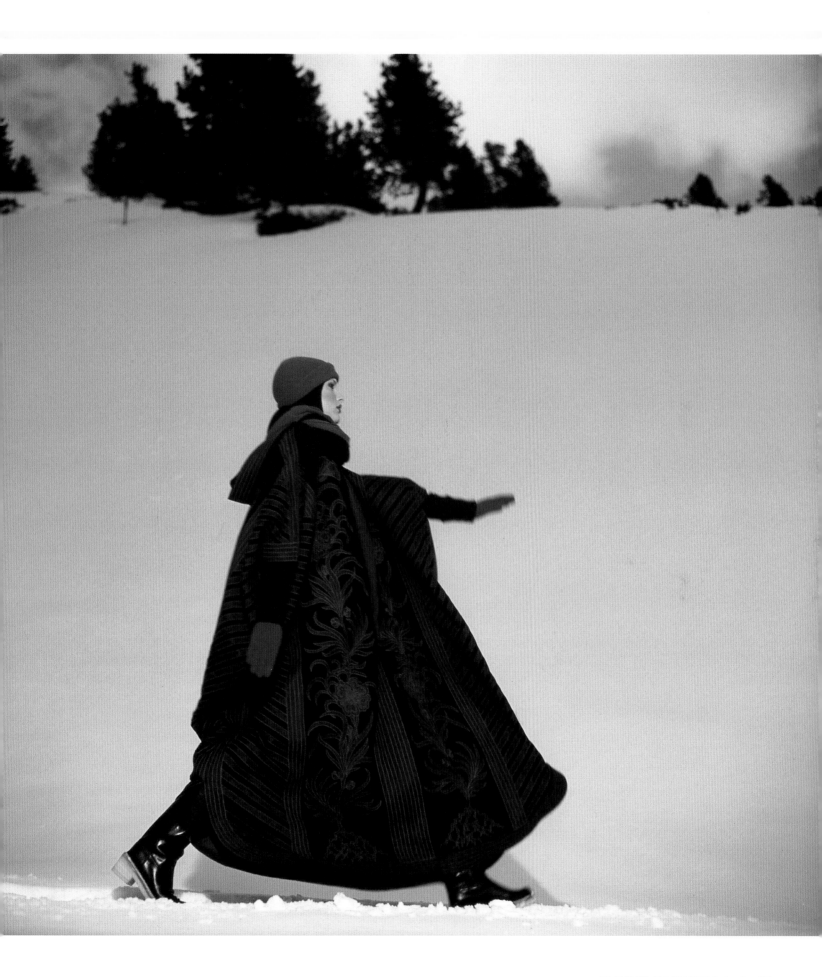

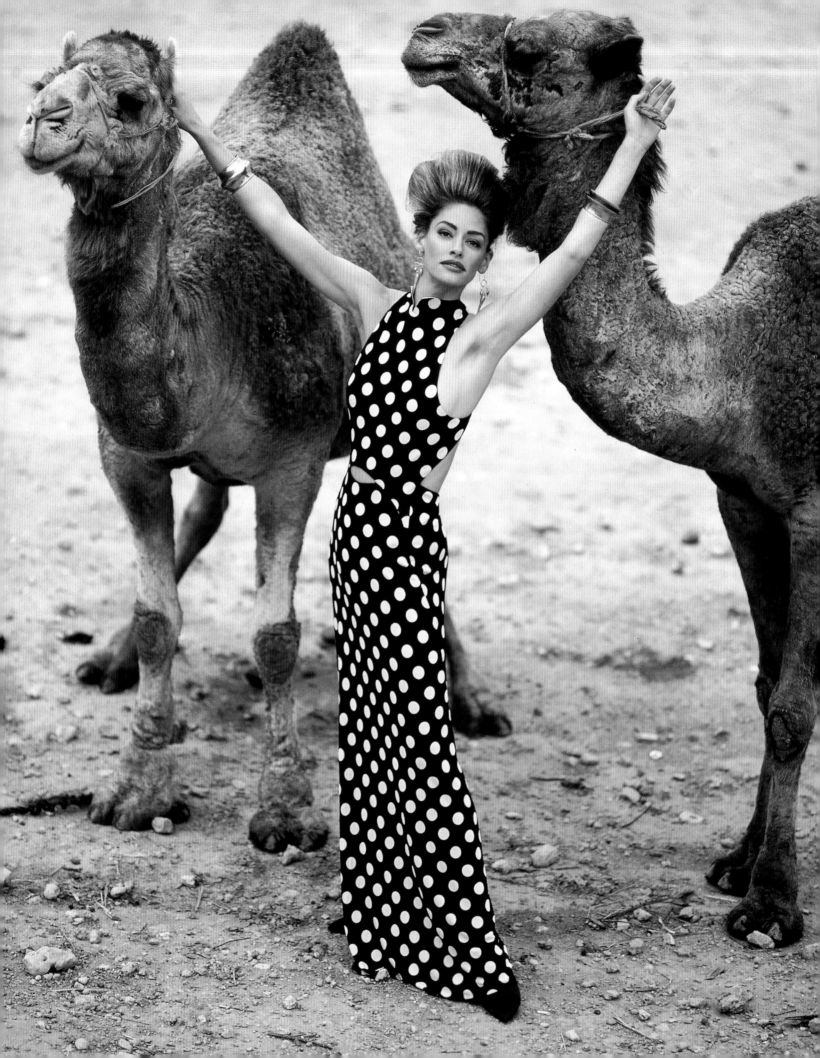

BEENE, Geoffrey

BORN: HAYNESVILLE, LOUISIANA, USA, 1927

A resolute modernist and designer's designer who works in a mixture of mediums, Geoffrey Beene is a quiet thinker with a soft southern accent, who calls his clothes 'liquid geometry'. Beene claims he did not leave but 'fled' Haynesville to study medicine at Tulane University in New Orleans and Los Angeles from 1943–6. He decided to switch to fashion after being mesmerized by Gilbert Adrian's designs for Joan Crawford in *Humoresque* (1946). Beene worked in the display department of the I Magnin store in Los Angeles and studied at Traphagan School of Fashion in New York before moving to Paris, where he studied at L'Académie Julian with a tailor who had worked with Edward Molyneux. In 1951 Beene left Paris, working with the designer Teal Traina before launching Geoffrey Beene Inc. in 1963.

Geoffrey Beene has always defied convention: in 1966 he was putting grey flannel and wool jersey into eveningwear, predicting jumpsuits would be the future of fashion and making sequinned sportswear. He launched Beenebag, one of America's first diffusion lines, in 1971. In 1976 he was the first American designer to show in Milan, prompting *L'Uomo Vogue* to issue a warning: 'Look out Italian designers. This is the future.' Beene was famously made *persona non grata* by buyer's bible *Women's Wear Daily* in 1967 – allegedly because he wouldn't give advance details of the wedding dress he had designed for Lynda Bird Johnson. 'I felt my allegiance was to the President,' he told *Vogue* in 1987. The ensuing feud lasted for decades. This would have been commercial suicide for most designers, but not for Beene, who survived with a hard-core clientele and a sense of humour: 'I've been called a lot of things other than Mr Beene, believe me.'

With eight Coty Awards under his belt, Beene has been both employer and mentor to some of the most talented American designers, including Gene Mayer, Alber Elbaz and Issey Miyake – Japan's forefather of aesthetic dressing. His talents are not confined to fashion. Beene also designs furniture, shoes and accessories, and has cultivated a collection of over 2,000 orchids. Despite being on the board of the American Ballet Theatre, he had never designed dance costumes until he was commissioned by Twyla Tharp Company for the 1999 dance work *Diabelli*.

Beene is one of fashion's thinkers, a revolutionary, a fabric technologist, who lives a solitary existence with two dachshunds. He hates looking back. 'The future of fashion is performance,' Beene told *Life*. 'Clothes will be packable, versatile and practically weightless. I said about 10 years ago that the major change in fashion will come about when the chemist meets with the artist.'

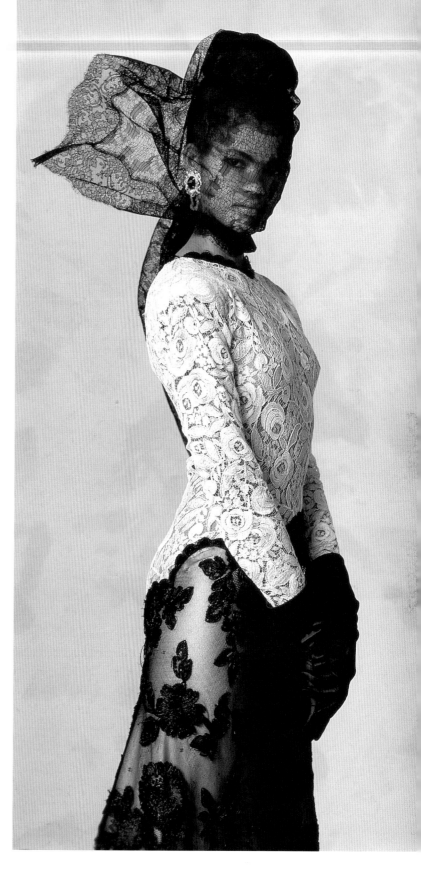

OPPOSITE **Master minimalist Beene's navy and white spotted evening dress in silk jersey with long bias-cut skirt, 1992.**

ABOVE **Cream corded and black embroidered lace come together in Beene's diagonal edge-to-edge scalloped evening dress, 1986.**

BENETTON

FOUNDED BY LUCIANO, GIULIANA, GILBERTO AND CARLO BENETTON IN 1965

The Italian knitwear company, Benetton, caused a stir by producing a series of shocking advertising campaigns directed by its creative director, Oliviero Toscani. Scenes splashed across billboards and magazines included an AIDS patient on his deathbed, and another of a baby complete with umbilical cord. Benetton claimed they were promoting social awareness, but critics pointed out that photojournalism had nothing to do with selling sweaters. Whatever the moral standpoint, Benetton have sustained a high profile and are one of the best-known Italian companies in the world.

BERARDI, Antonio

BORN: GRANTHAM, ENGLAND, 1968

Rising star Antonio Berardi told *Vogue* in 1997, 'My work is a mix of my British and Sicilian roots: an art school mentality combined with the inspiration I take from the strength of the women in my family.' Berardi, whose Sicilian parents owned an ice cream business, graduated from London's Central Saint Martins College of Art and Design in 1994, already showing signs of pulling power: his show featured hats by Philip Treacy and shoes by Manolo Blahnik; hairdresser Sam McKnight and make-up artist Mary Greenwell gave their services free of charge. In December 1996 Berardi signed up with Italian manufacturers Givuesse and in 1999 he showed for the first time in Italy. His collection, 'Never Mind the Borgias', contained punk and Renaissance references, his *pièce de résistance* a jacket constructed from 200 zips. Later that year he made matching purple outfits for the wedding of Victoria Adams (Posh Spice) to Manchester United star David Beckham – and their baby Brooklyn.

BIAGIOTTI, Laura

BORN: ROME, ITALY, 1943

With designs that are quiet, clean and spare, in classic fabrics and neutral colours, Laura Biagiotti has forged a reputation for understated Italian clothing that needs no concepts or gimmicks to sell it. Biagiotti studied literature and archaeology before returning to the family's ready-to-wear company in 1962. She worked with Roberto Cappuci and freelanced with a host of other Italian designers before founding her own label. Italian in thinking but international in attitude, the Laura Biagiotti label sells as far afield as Thailand, China and Moscow.

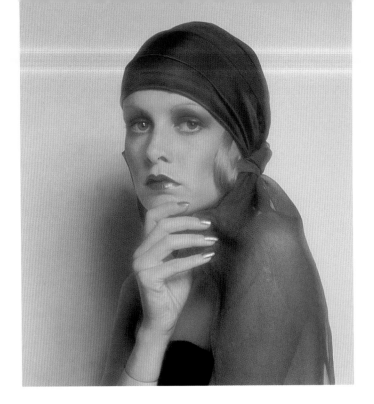

BIBA

FOUNDED BY BARBARA HULANICKI
BORN: WARSAW, POLAND, 1936

Barbara Hulanicki's biography, *From A to Biba* (1983), is dedicated 'To All Optimists, Fatalists and Dreamers', a fitting introduction to a story of extraordinary vision and retail invention, which captured the imagination of a generation. Biba was the parting shot of the 1960s: the seminal moment of shopping without cynicism.

Biba's creator, Barbara Hulanicki, started as a fashion artist and began Biba's Postal Boutique in the early 1960s. Her first dress – a gingham shift with matching headscarf – sold via the *Daily Mirror* for 25 shillings. The first Biba shop, formerly a small chemist's in Abingdon Road, Kensington, London, was opened in 1964. A series of publicity coups followed: Cathy McGowan, the hip presenter of the pop programme *Ready Steady Go*, wore a Biba smock dress on television, and Biba provided the wardrobe for the film *Darling* (1965), staring Julie Christie. Biba moved to bigger premises on Kensington High Street in 1969, and Hulanicki's ultimate dream came true in 1973 when the label took over the magnificent Derry and Toms department store – a huge Art Deco space with original fittings.

ABOVE 'Twiggy – plain Twiba – wearing Biba, that is' in 1973, showing off Biba's china doll foundation and femme fatale look to its best advantage.

OPPOSITE Twiggy in the entrance to Biba's extravagant changing rooms, wearing Biba's great spot trenchcoat with matching fake leopard pillbox hat, 1973.

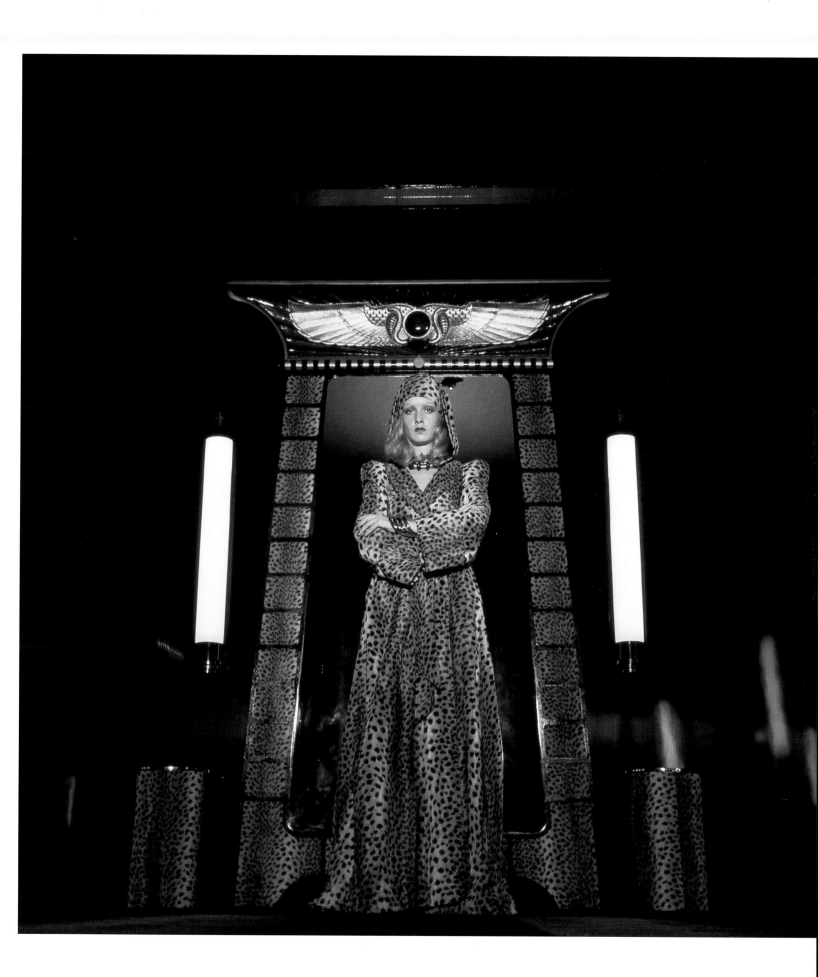

Hulanicki's attention to detail knew no bounds: Biba was an oasis of gorgeousness, where customers could buy tins of beans and feather boas, black and plum lipsticks, each with Biba's logo of lacquered black and swirling gold. A mesmerizing monument to Art Deco and Art Nouveau, the interior was described by *Vogue* in 1973 as 'a palace of apricot marble, coloured counters and fake leopardskin walls. Six floors of pure 1930s fantasy.' Although visually stunning, the venture was commercially unsound, the store too huge, the lighting too dark. Biba became a financial nightmare and a shoplifters' paradise. Declared bankrupt in 1976, Hulanicki moved to Brazil and then to Miami Beach, Florida, where she has turned her talent to designing hotels.

BIKKEMBERGS, Dirk

BORN: FLAMERSHEIM, GERMANY, 1962

Part of the Belgian contingent that gained prominence during the early 1990s, Dirk Bikkembergs first became famous for his footwear, with his functional, hard-wearing shoes.

Bikkembergs studied fashion at the Royal Academy of Arts in Antwerp, and worked as a freelance designer for a variety of companies before launching his own line in 1985. His first menswear collection was shown in 1988, followed by womenswear five years later.

BIRTWELL, Celia

BORN: BURY, ENGLAND, 1941

Depicted in countless canvases and drawings by David Hockney, Celia Birtwell is a talented textile designer and superb colourist, most famous for her electric collaborations with her late ex-husband, Ossie Clark. Both are immortalized in London's Tate Gallery's most popular portrait, *Mr and Mrs Clark and Percy*, painted by Hockney in 1970.

Celia – then a beatnik in winkle-picker shoes – met Ossie Clark via Mo McDermott in Manchester. She had been attending Salford Art School since the age of 13, eventually teaching cake decoration. Celia travelled south to London in 1962. She never went back.

Most famous for her extraordinary prints on silk chiffon, which she produced during her marriage to Ossie Clark, she now has her own shop in London's Westbourne Park Road and has a fabric collection called 'Celia's Stripes' to be launched by Zoffany in the millennium. Speaking in 1994 of her partnership with Ossie Clark, she said, 'We were marvellous together. A very peculiar, strange mix that was pretty powerful.'

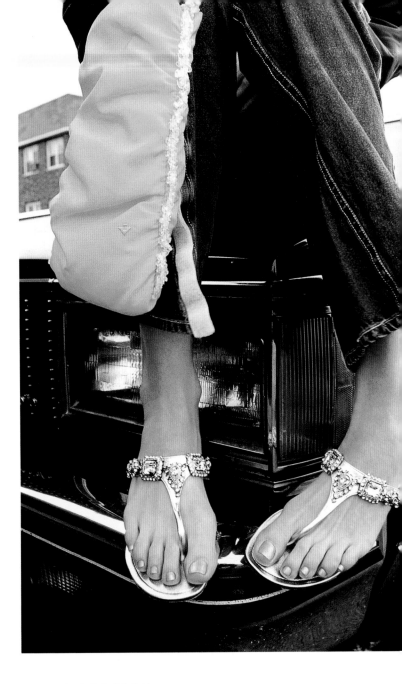

BLAHNIK, Manolo

BORN: SANTA CRUZ, CANARY ISLANDS, 1942

'If God had wanted women to wear flat shoes, he wouldn't have created Manolo Blahnik,' wrote *Vogue* editor Alexandra Shulman in July 1994. An Englishman with branches in New York and a home in Bath, Blahnik is a master shoemaker in a world of plummeting standards. Like most great designers, he follows his own line. He has a distinct aversion to platforms and predominantly uses silk and satin. 'Quality in everything is paramount,' he told *Vogue* in 1990.

Of Czech and Spanish parentage, Blahnik studied law, literature and Renaissance art at university in Geneva before moving to London in 1970. On showing his portfolio to *Vogue*, the then editor Diana Vreeland suggested that he concentrate on shoe designs, a proposal that played an instrumental part in his rise. He opened his first shop and called it Zapata, before reverting to his own name.

Blahnik's shoes are collected, cosseted and often regarded as being so exquisitely beautiful that they are put on display as works of art. He has been commissioned many times to design shoes for the collections of John Galliano, Isaac Mizrahi, Todd Oldham, Bill Blass and Alexander McQueen, among others. Lucy Ferry, wife of rock star Bryan, told *Vogue* in 1990, 'I bought my first pair in 1976 when I was sixteen and I've been buying them ever since. Other shoemakers don't have his imagination, or the incredible detail – such teeny weeny buckles, they're all perfect.'

BLASS, Bill

BORN: FORT WAYNE, INDIANA, USA, 1922

Bill Blass possesses the three key ingredients of a successful American designer: a good eye for design, a shrewd business brain and a personality that charms the birds off the trees. His talent for licensing is legendary: Blassport sportswear was launched in 1972 and his signature perfume in 1978; other products include swimwear, jeans, bedlinen and shoes.

Blass came to New York when he was 17 years old and spent a brief spell as a sketch artist before becoming a sergeant in the army. He designed at Anna Miller and Company, New York, and then moved on to Seventh Avenue's Maurice Retner, where he was so successful that his was one of the first American designer's names to appear on the label. On Retner's retirement, Blass became the owner and in 1973 Bill Blass Limited was born.

Blass has won countless awards including the Coty American Fashion Critics' Award, which he has won three times, and the Gentlemen's Quarterly Award in 1981. On 25 May 1999 he received the first Lifetime Achievement Award from the Fashion Institute of Technology. He holds three Honorary Doctorate degrees and was one of the founder members of the Council of Fashion Designers of America (CFDA). President Reagan appointed Blass to the President's Committee on the Arts and Humanities in 1987. In January 1994 he contributed $10 million to the New York Public Library, which now has a public reading room in his name.

OPPOSITE **The maestro of the high heel, Manolo Blahnik, switches to flat thong sandals in 1999, made from a mix of diamanté and silver leather.**

RIGHT **Bill Blass's 'brilliant stem of cyclamen and yellow silk crepe' of 1986, with a sweeping skirt and a bodice cut to resemble a bolero.**

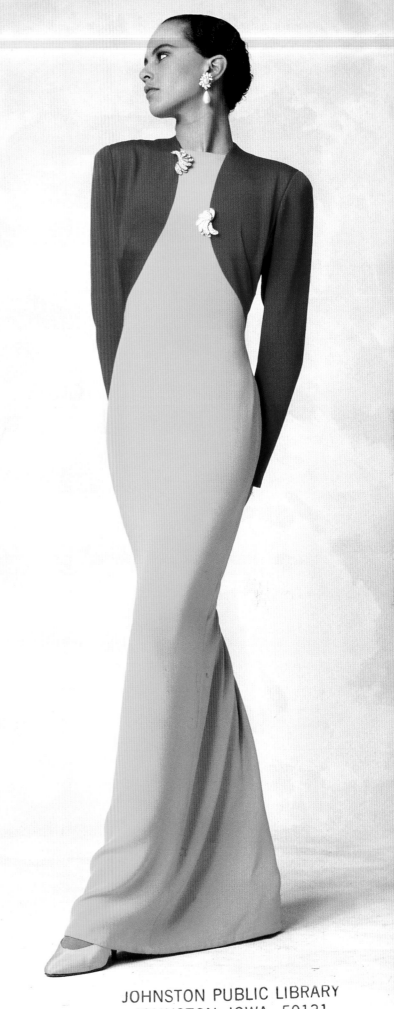

BODYMAP

FOUNDED BY DAVID HOLAH AND STEVIE STEWART IN 1982

'Young designers are re-drawing the hemline, any line, and not always with a ruler,' said *Vogue* in its assessment of the new cotton softwear in 1984. Bodymap were a breath of fresh air in the early 1980s, mixing stretch forms, ribbing and graphic patterns by textile designer Hilde Smith.

Holah and Stewart met at Middlesex Polytechnic, progressed to a stall in Camden Market and graduated with first-class honours. Heavily influenced by the Japanese avant-garde and Vivienne Westwood, their 1984 show, with its bare breasts and skullcaps, prompted the *Daily News Record* to question whether it was 'an outrageous pretension or merely a pretentious outrage'. The press went crazy. Buyers bought in droves. Bodymap held a 'Survival in the Fashion World' party in 1989. Unfortunately, what it really needed was a creative accountant and sympathetic backer – the business folded in 1991.

BOHAN, Marc

BORN: PARIS, FRANCE, 1926

'Marc Bohan is small, dark and quicksilver, and a most sophisticated man as befitting the artistic director of Christian Dior, the house that spells the ultimate in luxury for perhaps the greatest number of people in the world,' said *Vogue* in 'The Perfectionists' in 1974.

Bohan has a meticulous design pedigree: he worked at Jean Patou in 1945, Robert Piquet in 1946 and Edward Molyneux in 1950, returning to Patou in 1953 as designer of the haute couture collections. In 1958 Bohan spent time in America, familiarizing himself with Seventh Avenue. He prepared and designed the Christian Dior London collections in 1958, and in September 1960 he travelled to England to create their ready-to-wear collections. In 1960, on his appointment as artistic director at Christian Dior,

Bohan returned to Paris, where he continued to produce immaculate collections for Dior until 1989. In 1990 Bohan was persuaded to return to London to Hartnell, which had been floundering since its founder's death. Although Bohan's collections were well received, financial difficulties and lack of licensing income meant Hartnell had to close. On his appointment at Hartnell, Bohan recalled Molyneux's advice, which he had adhered to all his life: 'Amuse yourself with sketches, not with dresses.'

BOUÉ SŒURS, House of

FOUNDED BY SYLVIE AND JEANNE BOUÉ IN 1899

'Two fairy aprons float upon the skirt in front and back ... Add sparkle, and faint motion.' *Vogue*'s lyrical description of Boué Sœurs dresses captured the ethereal quality of one of the most distinctive signatures of the century. Boué Sœurs – two sisters who had a common love of embellishment – crossed the line between lingerie and outerwear. Using theatrical, iridescent fabrics with light-reflective surfaces, silver and gold lace trimming, ribbons, translucent fabrics and pale colours, Boué Sœurs made dresses with a wistful quality. Frequent visitors to America, Boué Sœurs, like Callot Sœurs, had a loyal transatlantic following. By the 1930s, when fashion fell out with surface effects, the Boué Sœurs ceased to exist.

BRUCE, Liza

BORN: NEW YORK, USA, 1955

Liza Bruce built her business on stretch fabric and quickly became known as the 'Queen of Lycra', producing swimsuits of the neon-coloured variety, aerodynamic lines and cut-outs. With no formal training and a foray into the restaurant business, Bruce progressed from swimsuits into catsuits and curvy dresses. Interviewed by *Vogue* in 1990 she said, 'Posture is central to looking youthful and, as clothes become more streamlined, good posture will become even more important.'

BURBERRY

FOUNDED BY THOMAS BURBERRY IN 1856

An inventor and fabric technologist, who predicted the advent of sportswear and steered its course, Thomas Burberry opened his shop in Basingstoke, Hampshire, in 1856 when he was 21 years old. In 1888 he took out a patent for improved materials and was making waterproof garments by the turn of the century.

In 1901 Burberry designed clothes for the new leisured classes, sportswear and the utility raincoat – the famous Burberry check originated in Edinburgh in 1924, but became hot property in the 1960s. He also designed a new service uniform for British officers and Sir Ernest Shackleton's Outrig suit, worn on the British Everest Expedition of 1924.

The classic Burberry trenchcoat is recognized all over the world and has appeared many times on film including *Torn Curtain* (1966), *Kramer Versus Kramer* (1979), *Wall Street* (1987), *Dick Tracy* (1990) and *The Pink Panther Strikes Again* (1976), during the filming of which Peter Sellers always had two on set. Marcello Mastroianni used the classic trench in all his films during the 1950s and 1960s. Celebrity wearers included Grace Kelly, Ingrid Bergman and Jacques Tati.

Backed by an advertising campaign photographed by Mario Testino, the Burberry flagship store, at 18–22 Haymarket, London, has recently been beautifully revamped under the direction of Rose Marie Bravo, formerly of Manhattan's Saks Fifth Avenue, who was appointed worldwide chief executive of Burberry in October 1997. The following February Roberto Menichetti, who previously worked for both Claude Montana and Jil Sander, was appointed creative director.

BURROWS, Stephen

BORN: NEWARK, NEW JERSEY, USA, 1943

Best known for his use of colour, Stephen Burrows' career has fluctuated as many times as his styles. He studied at New York's Fashion Institute of Technology and spent two years working in New York's fashion industry. Picked up and promoted relentlessly by Henri Bendel department store in the 1970s, he was given his own in-store boutique called Stephen Burrows' World. Frequently in and out of fashion, Burrows' clothes have a wide appeal and have been worn by Debbie Harry of Blondie and Diana Ross.

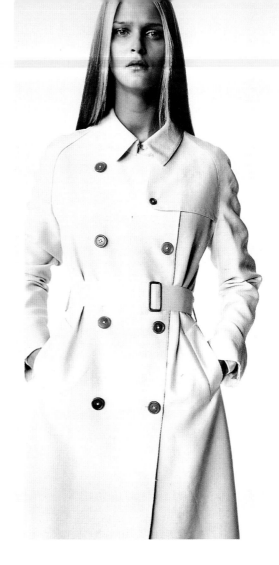

BYBLOS

FOUNDED IN 1973

A company which previously employed Gianni Versace and Guy Paulin as its in-house designers, Byblos was successfully directed from 1981 by Keith Varty and Alan Cleaver. Known as the 'Byblos boys', Varty and Cleaver are both English designers who totally understand the Italian sensibility. 'A company like Byblos simply doesn't exist in England,' they told *Vogue* in 1990. 'We don't have a budget – nobody questions how much we spend on fabrics. Coming to Italy opened our eyes to the importance of quality. The British have a whole different sense of priorities. In Italy, designers are treated like pop stars.' Byblos made Richard Tyler design director in 1999, followed by John Bartlett.

OPPOSITE **Riding on the wave of unconventional cutting, Bodymap's pattern, stretch and a fish fin skirt: textiles by Hilde Smith, 1986.**

ABOVE **Still wowing the raincoat devotees, Burberry 1999-style. Knee-length mac with functional detail, but made in silk, by Burberry Prorsum.**

CACHAREL, Jean

BORN: NÎMES, FRANCE, 1932

Originally a men's tailor, Jean Cacharel switched to womenswear when he became a pattern cutter and stylist at Jean Jourdan of Paris. He founded his own business at the turn of the 1960s, perfectly capturing the downturn of couture and upward mobility of ready to wear. Cacharel sealed his fame when he collaborated with Liberty of London during the mid-1960s, revamping their traditional prints and making them relevant to a hipper, younger clientele. The Cacharel label consequently became synonymous with sporty, easy shapes, adding childrenswear, jeans and menswear in 1994, and two phenomenally successful fragrances – Anais Anais and Lou Lou. Jean Cacharel received an Export Trade Oscar in 1969.

CALLOT SŒURS, House of

FOUNDED BY SISTERS GERBER, BERTRAND AND CHANTERELLE IN 1895

Exotic and breathtakingly beautiful dresses bearing the Callot Sœurs label still astound. Like their creators, they have an air of mystique. 'A curious situation controls the house of Callot. Its gowns are known wherever smart gowns are worn, yet the women who govern the house are almost mythical. It would be a mockery to apply the word "fashionable" to these women: they would despise it. They never go out at all,' said *Vogue* in 1915. Previously in business separately, the reclusive Callot sisters decided to pool their resources, eventually moving to the avenue Matignon, Paris, employing 1,500 workers and supplying a huge American market. The Callot Sœurs were world authorities on antique lace and were often called upon for advice by French and foreign museums. *Vogue* imbued the sisters with a legendary sense of mystery: 'Silently, working away with their shears and thread, they weave

LEFT 'A graceful arrangement of floating red tulle edged with black chantilly' by Callot Sœurs, worn by Miss Elsie de Wolfe at a dance given by Madame Hyde, 1920.

clothes that bring them millions, and from their workroom, into which no stranger penetrates, they govern the destiny of continents they have not seen.'

CAPELLINO, Ally

BORN: HAMPTON COURT, ENGLAND, 1956

Modern, easy and eternally wearable, Ally Capellino's brand of English simplicity has worldwide appeal. Alison Lloyd – the designer behind the Ally Capellino label – graduated from Middlesex Polytechnic in fashion and textiles in 1978, and worked at the Courtauld Institute in London before forming her own company selling accessories, millinery and jewellery in 1979. She established the Ally Capellino label the following year. In addition to producing collections, being involved in Crafts Council projects and design consultancy work, Ally lectures at the Royal College of Art and Central Saint Martins College of Art and Design in London, passing on her expertise to stars of the future.

CAPUCCI, Roberto

BORN: ROME, ITALY, 1929

An expert in sculptural shape and circular form, Roberto Capucci was one of the first post-Second World War Italian couturiers to enjoy international fame. In 1961 *Vogue* described Capucci's crisp, abbreviated shift: 'Nothing more than stark, elegant shapes with hems cropped daringly short – designed to make women look outrageously young yet *mondaine*.'

After spending a decade designing in Rome, Capucci moved to Paris with the backing of a Florentine businessman and opened his own salon on rue Cambon. He returned to Rome six years later to resume his experimentalism and open another salon on Via Gregoriana. Capucci's designs are not just about his use of fabric; he has also incorporated ribbons, pebbles and quilting to enhance his organic forms.

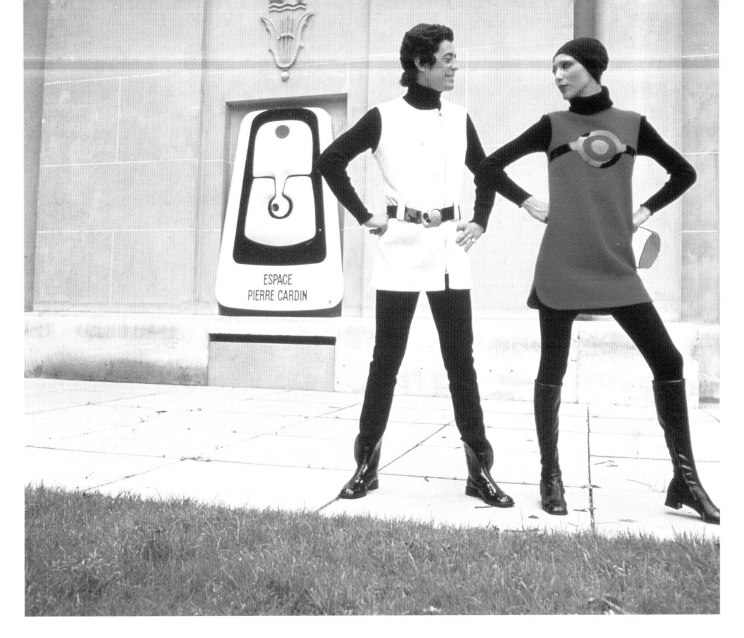

CARDIN, Pierre

BORN: SAN ANDREA DA BARBARA, ITALY, 1922

In 1974 *Vogue*'s assessment of Pierre Cardin was as a 'ferbrile, anguished, original, the air quaking about him as he hurtles from place to place, project to project.' The cover of *Forbes* magazine 15 years later was emblazoned with the words, 'Pierre Cardin: Why am I bad if I sell a frying pan?' For Pierre Cardin, read: paradox. Visionary designer and unashamed licencee.

Cardin's career began as a tailor's cutter in Vichy, France. He opened his own business in 1950, with his first haute couture collection in 1953 and a boutique the following year. Cardin personified the forward-thinking 1960s with his preoccupation with science fiction: jumpsuits and plastic discs; helmets instead of hats. With a marketing strategy years ahead of its time, Cardin extended the tentacles of his empire into new territory, pre-empting the mass-market explosion of the 1960s. In 1956 he was the first European designer to establish himself in Japan, and in 1981 he was the first to open a showroom in China. He has been saying since the 1960s that he would like to have the first boutique on the moon.

With 840 licences in 125 countries, the world-famous Cardin name has appeared on a variety of products – from furniture to private jets, chocolates to nuts. Cardin told *Vogue* in 1990, 'After those, of course, they all sneered and said I'd be doing sardine tins next, and I said why not? It's all part of the creative process.'

ABOVE **Space-age 'cosmos' creations by Pierre Cardin. Models pose – 1966-style – in front of Cardin's L'Espace.**

CARNEGIE, Hattie

BORN: VIENNA, AUSTRIA, 1889
DIED: NEW YORK, NEW YORK, USA, 1956

The first American designer to make the psychological leap between design and lifestyle, Hattie Carnegie was a retail phenomena who imported Paris couture into America – sometimes diluting the styles under the Hattie Carnegie Originals label. The Carnegie headquarters on East 49th Street stocked jewellery, cosmetics, sportswear – even antiques and Carnegie chocolates.

Carnegie's forceful and opinionated nature was legendary. She was an astute businesswoman with a sharp commercial brain, who began her career as a trainee milliner and runner at Macy's. In 1909 she opened a hat and dress shop on East 10th Street. Carnegie specialized in the complete look – advising and providing everything from gloves to cosmetics. After her death in 1956, the company carried on, but when fashion swung in favour of the adolescent, the Carnegie business – inextricably linked with its creator – went to the wall.

CASHIN, Bonnie

BORN: OAKLAND, CALIFORNIA, USA, 1915

Years ahead of her time, Bonnie Cashin was both an innovator and experimentalist. In the mid-1930s she became costume designer for Manhattan's Roxy Theatre, where she learnt the principles of movement and shape. Spotted by sportswear supremo Louis Adler, Cashin designed for his company, Adler and Adler, for over a decade. In 1953 she reverted to the freelance lifestyle. While the silhouette of the 1950s dictated cinched waists and tight fits, Cashin stayed true to her principles of modernity and purity. Her timeless shapes, based on triangles, rectangles and squares, formed the foundation of American fashion in the twentieth century.

CASSINI, Oleg

BORN: PARIS, FRANCE, 1913

A renowned Casanova and professional charmer, Oleg Cassini is a Russian count who is famous for three things: his pencilled moustache, his engagement to Grace Kelly and the official wardrobe he designed for the century's most elegant first lady, Jacqueline Kennedy.

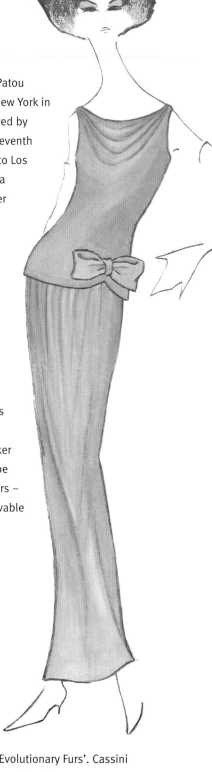

Cassini trained at Jean Patou in Paris, before moving to New York in 1936, where he was employed by various manufacturers on Seventh Avenue. In 1940 he moved to Los Angeles, where he became a Hollywood costume designer under Edith Head. He also dated a number of starlets, before deciding to settle down with actress Gene Tierney. By 1950, Cassini was back on Seventh Avenue – where his name became synonymous with glamorous sheath dresses, knitted jackets and cocktail dresses. In 1961 Cassini was appointed Jacqueline Kennedy's official dressmaker and formulated her wardrobe during her White House years – from a wool coat with removable collar of Russian sable to the A-line dress at the Pre-Inaugural Gala, which Cassini described in 1991 as 'audacious, studied simplicity'.

In 1961 Cassini made a leopardskin fur coat for Jacqueline Kennedy. Almost 40 years later, he attempted to redress the balance with a fake fur collection called 'Evolutionary Furs'. Cassini told *The Sunday Times* in 1999, 'Fashion is not couture anymore. It is show business.' At 86 years old, Cassini's pencilled moustache was still intact.

ABOVE **'Mrs Kennedy's New Evening Choices'** – an ankle-length evening dress of green silk jersey created by Oleg Cassini in 1961 for America's first lady.

OPPOSITE **Bonnie Cashin's 'high voltage coat and dress'.** A shocking-red kidskin coat, ruffled in racoon and lined in fleece, photographed by Helmut Newton, 1966.

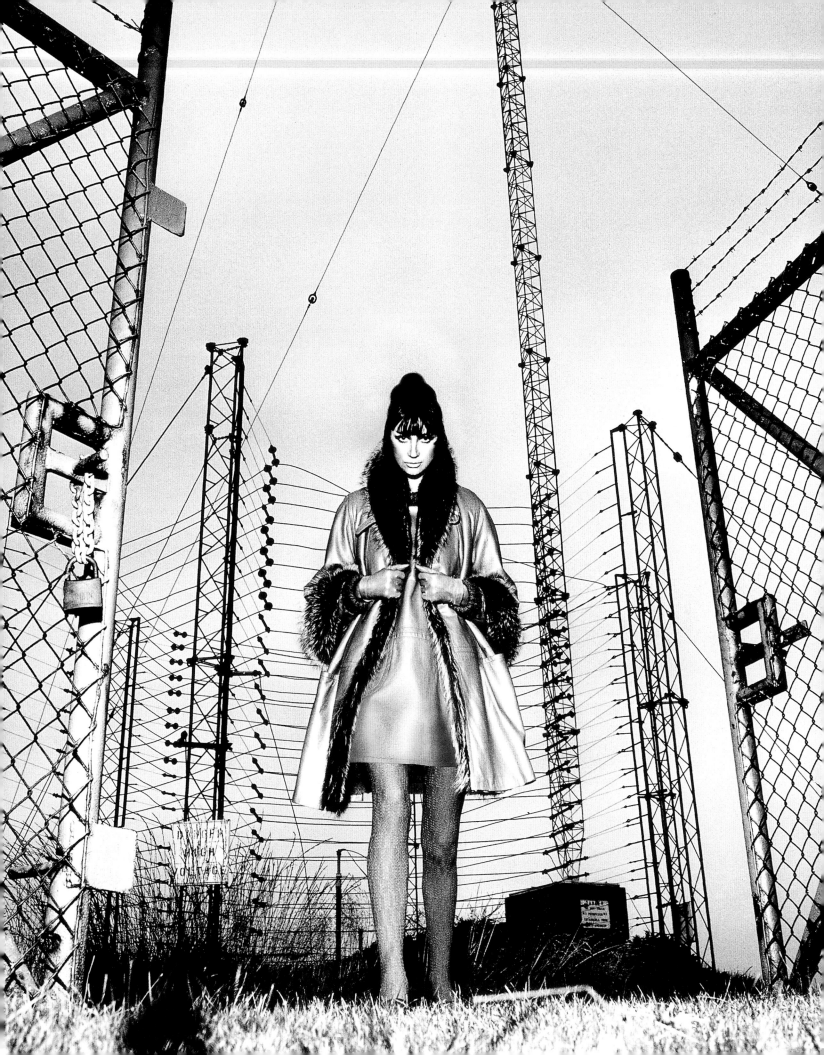

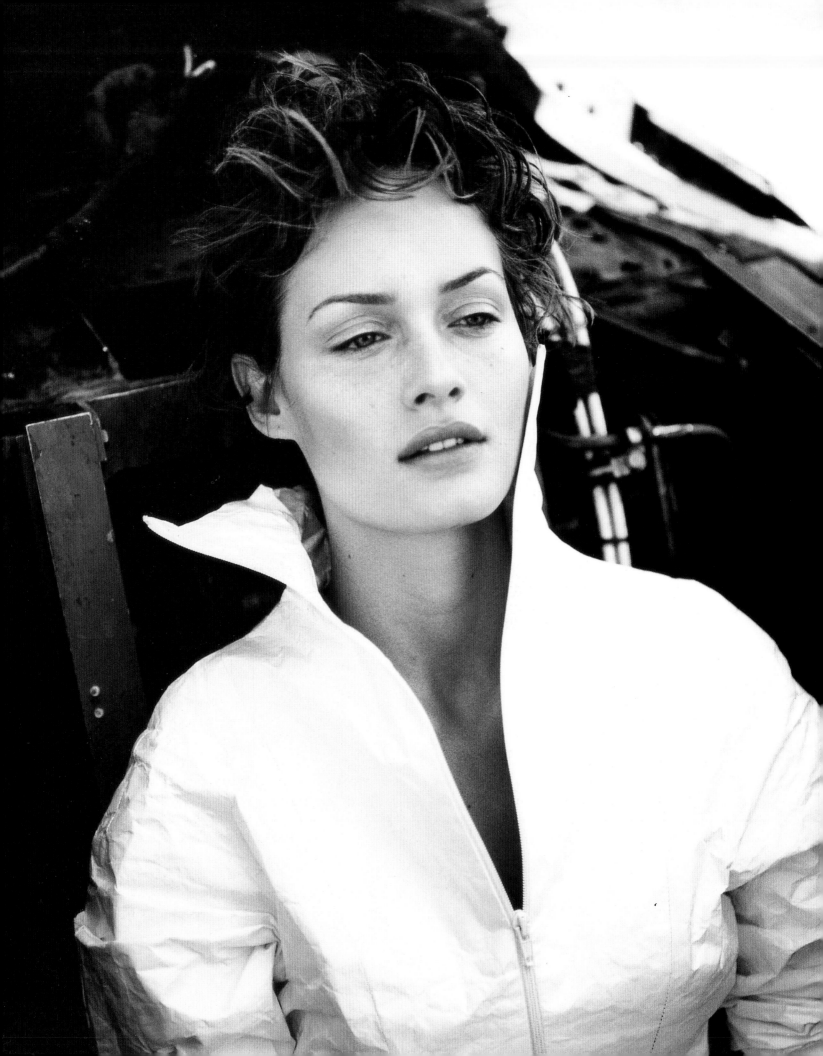

CASTELBAJAC,
Jean-Charles de

BORN: CASABLANCA, MOROCCO, 1949

With his flair for architectural shapes and clear blocks of colour, Jean-Charles de Castelbajac has always been associated with streamlined design. He formed a ready-to-wear fashion company with his mother and freelanced for various companies from Max Mara to Levi Strauss. In 1970 he launched his own label and his collections have been exhibited in Paris, Austria and Belgium. In addition, Castelbajac has designed for film and stage, including the pop group Talking Heads. In 1979 he began designing furniture and interiors. For two years he designed the collections of André Courrèges, the 1960s' designer who epitomized futurism.

CAVANAGH, John

BORN: IRELAND, 1914

A former assistant to Edward Molyneux and, briefly, Pierre Balmain, John Cavanagh opened his London salon in 1952. *Vogue* summed up his style with a description of his customers: 'His clients move with the times in an establishment world: their kind of life ranges from the country weekend to jet propelled globetrotting.' He is a member of the Incorporated Society of London Fashion Designers, together with London luminaries Norman Hartnell, Digby Morton and Lachasse. Cavanagh designed the wedding dresses for both the Duchess of Kent and Princess Alexandra.

CÉLINE

FOUNDED IN 1973

Céline is a French luxury brand which was founded in 1973 but did not make its mark until two years later when the first Céline boutiques opened around the world: starting with Monte Carlo, Geneva and Hong Kong, followed by London, Toronto and Beverly Hills. Sponsoring the French Open and America's Cup in the 1980s raised Céline's profile.

OPPOSITE **One of Hussein Chalayan's early pieces, 1994: a modern zip-up 'paper' jacket with elongated collar – 'unrippable and washable.'**

In 1997 Michael Kors was appointed chief ready-to-wear designer. The first collection was a resounding success – a sea of calm, quiet colours – and, although Kors had produced the show in double-quick time, he remained – like the clothes – cool, calm and collected. Kors now holds the position of creative director.

CERRUTI, Nino

BORN: BIELLA, ITALY, 1930

Probably most famous for his menswear, Nino Cerruti took over his family's textile business at 20 years old and produced his own line in 1957. His early collections were considered avant-garde and revolutionary. Later, he became a consummate businessman, paring down and refining his designs for the mass-market. He started his career creating hip menswear, progressed into knitwear, unisex in 1967 and womenswear in 1976. Like Giorgio Armani, Cerruti rarely wavers from his principles, preferring clean, restrained tailoring.

CHALAYAN, Hussein

BORN: NICOSIA, CYPRUS, 1970

More fine artist than fashion designer, Hussein Chalayan has broken the mould of British fashion by being a quiet minimalist as opposed to rebel without a cause. He is the only British designer to compete intellectually with Comme des Garçons.

Chalayan graduated from Central Saint Martins College of Art and Design in London in 1993 with a first-class honours degree and final collection entitled 'The Tangent Flows'. Armed with an envelope of metal filings and fabric buried in his back garden, his unconventional approach brought a commission from the equally unconventional Icelandic singer, Björk.

An intense thinker, who isn't part of the fashion circuit, Chalayan's main concession to commercialism is a capsule high street collection and a contract with New York cashmere company, TSE. His experimental ideas – the wooden corset, the moulded dress with armrest – are counterpointed by his pliable paper clothes. His designs – best analysed in depth and from all sides – suit the art installation approach: he has exhibited in Paris, Prague and at London's Science Museum. Awarded British Designer of the Year in March 1999, it is a pity Chalayan cannot experiment with shape and form to his heart's content. Fittingly, he constructed a plastic mechanical dress with designer Paul Topen to feature in London's Millennium Dome.

CHANEL, Gabrielle 'Coco'

Born: Saumur, France, 1883
Died: Paris, France, 1971

'Chanel is the fascinating paradox,' said *Vogue* in 1957, 'the couturier who takes no account of fashion, who pursues her own faultlessly elegant line in the quiet confidence that fashion will come back to her – and sure enough it always does.' The most influential designer of the twentieth century was a non-conformist with a classical streak. Coco Chanel designed the definitive women's suit, wore masculine clothes, sported a cropped haircut and flaunted a suntan when it was considered to be an emblem of the working classes. In 1916 she outraged the fashion industry by using jersey at a time when it was strictly associated with underwear. 'This designer made jersey what it is today – we hope she's satisfied,' snapped *Vogue* in 1917. 'It's almost as much part of our lives as blue serge is.' Modernity and comfort came naturally to Chanel. This was the key reason why the classic Chanel suit – collarless, simply cut, trimmed with braid and with a discreet chain sewn into the hem – has transcended every single movement of the twentieth century. 'Men make dresses in which one can't move,' she observed. 'They tell you very calmly that dresses aren't made for action.' Coco Chanel had a disappointing love life and brittle personality. She continually criticized her contemporaries: dismissing Elsa Schiaparelli as a dressmaker, accusing Christian Dior of dressing women like armchairs, and giving Cristobal Balenciaga the ultimate backhanded compliment in admiring his design, but questioning his ability to cut.

The first Chanel shop opened in Paris in 1914; by 1930 annual turnover totalled 120 million francs. When war broke out,

Chanel's salon on rue Cambon closed and she went into exile. When the salon reopened in 1954, Chanel was interviewed by *Vogue*. Now almost 70 years old, she was in a defiant mood: 'Look at today's dresses: strapless evening dresses cutting across a woman's front like this. Nothing is uglier for a woman; boned horrors, that's what they are.' On plagiarism: 'I have always been copied by others. If a fashion isn't taken up and worn by everybody, it's not a fashion but an eccentricity, a fancy dress.'

By 1969 Chanel had appeared consistently in *Vogue* for over 50 years.

Her place in history was secured. Already a legend, she was immortalized on Broadway in Alan Jay Lerner's musical *Coco*, which centred on Chanel's 1953–4 comeback; the lead role was played by Katharine Hepburn and the costumes were by Cecil Beaton, who received a coveted Tony Award for them. In her twilight years, Chanel lived a solitary existence, residing at the Ritz hotel in Paris.

The Chanel label found its natural successor, Karl Lagerfeld, in 1983. Lagerfeld's singular ability to astound, exploit and amuse – often all at the same time – took Chanel to the limit. His arrival coincided perfectly with the mood of the moment: a decade when conspicuous consumption and designer labels became the new religion.

LEFT 'This year's Chanel suit' – in 1957 – 'widely-ribbed navy blue jersey, fastening high with brass buttons, skirt features Chanel's new side pleat.'

OPPOSITE The Chanel suit, 1995 – collarless, trimmed in navy, and worn with a side zip miniskirt and sailor hat, modelled by Stella Tennant.

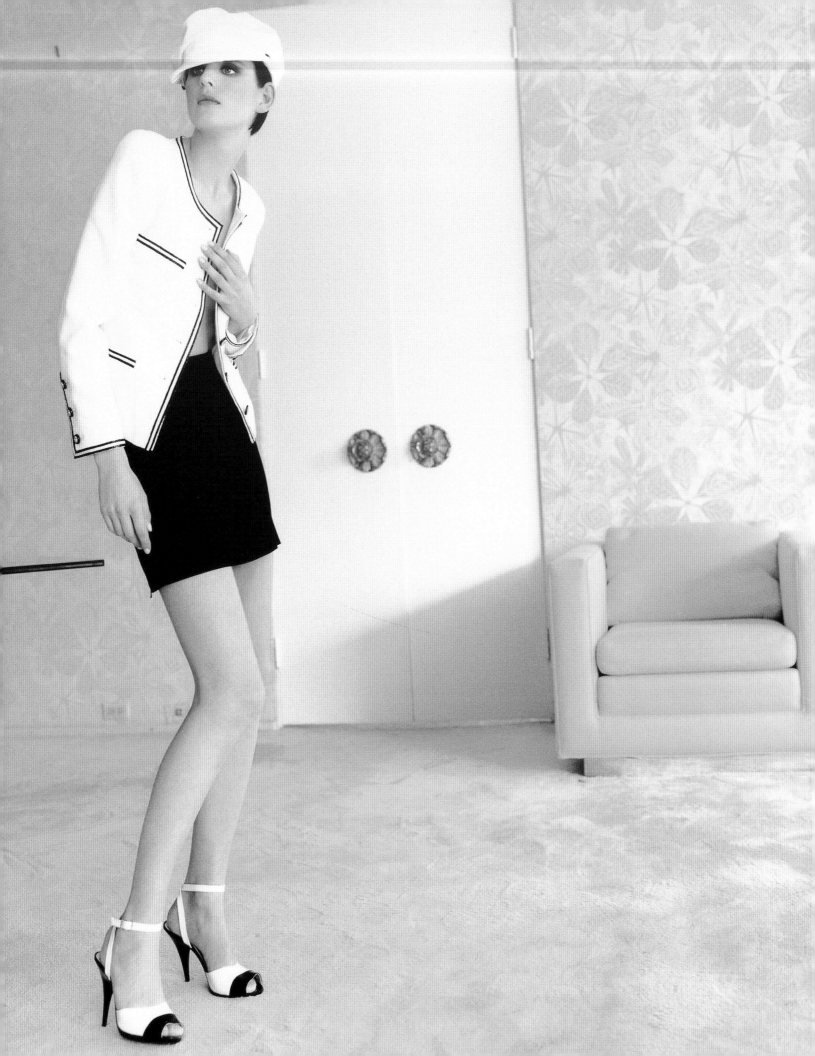

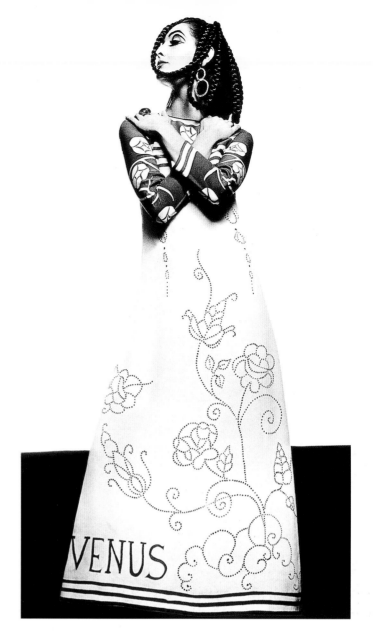

'Deep iris blue on white with flowers whirling straight from Tannhauser', a dramatic, exotic design from Chloé, 1967.

CHÉRUIT, Madeleine

FOUNDED BY MADELEINE CHÉRUIT IN 1900

Madeleine Chéruit was described in *Vogue* in 1915 as 'a Louis XVI woman because she has the daintiness, the extravagant tastes, the exquisite charm, and the art of those French ladies who went gaily through the pre-revolution epoch.' The house, designed by the architect Pierre Bullet and built in the early eighteenth century, extended from the place Vendôme to the rue des Petits-Champs. By 1915 the house of Chéruit was the property of Mesdames Wormser and Boulanger, who, *Vogue* observed in 1915, 'keep the house to its original type but bring much originality to it'. Apart from gowns, Chéruit was famous for its evening wraps, work in fur, children's clothes, lingerie, blouses and trousseaus.

CHLOÉ

FOUNDED BY GABY AGHION AND JACQUES LANOIR IN 1952

The Chloé philosophy of embodying young, forward-thinking design has always been reflected by the designers in Chloé's employ – Karl Lagerfeld, who worked at the company for almost 20 years, from 1965–83, again joining the company briefly in 1992; Martine Sitbon from 1987–91 before the appointment of Central Saint Martins College of Art and Design graduate, Stella McCartney. Her appointment, almost straight out of college, prompted shouts of nepotism. McCartney has proved she can deliver: the shows have been well received, sales figures are up and the Chloé look has a new, fresh perspective.

CHOO, Jimmy

BORN: PENANG, MALAYSIA, 1961

A relative newcomer to London's footwear fraternity – who established himself within the space of a decade – Jimmy Choo has shod a variety of the rich and famous. His clients included Diana, Princess of Wales, who had countless pairs of his high heels and flat pumps in her wardrobe.

Choo has gained a higher profile since the appointment of Tamara Yeardye, professional It Girl and managing director of the

company, who has helped his name become known on both sides of the Atlantic. Today, Jimmy Choo has branches in London, New York, Beverly Hills and Las Vegas. The first menswear collection was launched in February 1999.

CLAIBORNE, Liz

BORN: BRUSSELS, BELGIUM, 1929

Based on accessibility, versatility and quality, the Liz Claiborne label is revered and admired in corporate circles. The sheer size is astounding. Liz Claiborne studied fine art in Belgium and Nice, before finding her way into the fashion industry via illustration and a spell on New York's Seventh Avenue, eventually forming her own company in 1976.

Claiborne's success is built on divisions and a design appeal that has caught the imagination of the American public.

CLARK, Ossie

BORN: LIVERPOOL, ENGLAND, 1942
DIED: LONDON, ENGLAND, 1996

A genius cutter and constructor of clothes, Ossie Clark was the 1960s' wunderkind with all the essential ingredients: good looks, an extraordinary eye, an enormous ego and a talent to amuse. His bons mots littered the fashion pages of the 1960s and 1970s. The little black dress he christened 'a history of nice times'.

Ossie's ambiguous sexuality and instinctive feel for the female anatomy was at the core of his unique talent. He remains one of the few male fashion designers of the century who instinctively understood how women's bodies actually worked. 'His clothes were never vulgar,' said his ex-wife, textile designer Celia Birtwell, who he dressed during her two pregnancies with their sons Albert and George, 'I think he had respect for women. They were his goddesses.'

Ossie Clark was the product of a poor working-class family – the youngest of six children, who were evacuated to Oswaldtwistle during the Second World War. Encouraged by a schoolteacher who brought in glossy magazines, Ossie studied building, geometry and construction at Warrington Technical College, and in 1957 attended the Regional College of Art in Manchester. An outstanding talent, he secured a scholarship at London's Royal College of Art and emerged in 1965 with a first-class honours degree and a full page in *Vogue*. His final college collection featured graphic fabric, acquired during a drive across America with David Hockney in the summer of 1964.

A collaboration with Alice Pollock of Quorum in Chelsea's Radnor Walk catapulted Ossie Clark onto centre stage. Soon he was at the epicentre of the swinging sixties – friends included Patrick Procktor, David Hockney and Jimi Hendrix. Cecil Beaton attended his shows – along with London's glitterati. In 1966 Ossie married Celia Birtwell, who he met while she was teaching at Salford School of Art.

The magical meeting of Celia's textiles and Ossie's cutting created some of the most beautiful dresses of the decade – with plunging necklines, flowing sleeves and ethereal silhouettes. This was sensual perfection for the beautiful people. 'Ossie Clark's collection was a fantasy of the finest silks, cut velvet and dotted chiffon,' reported *Vogue* in 1971. 'The French were amazed and amused by the crazy glamour of Gala Mitchell, Ossie's London girl.'

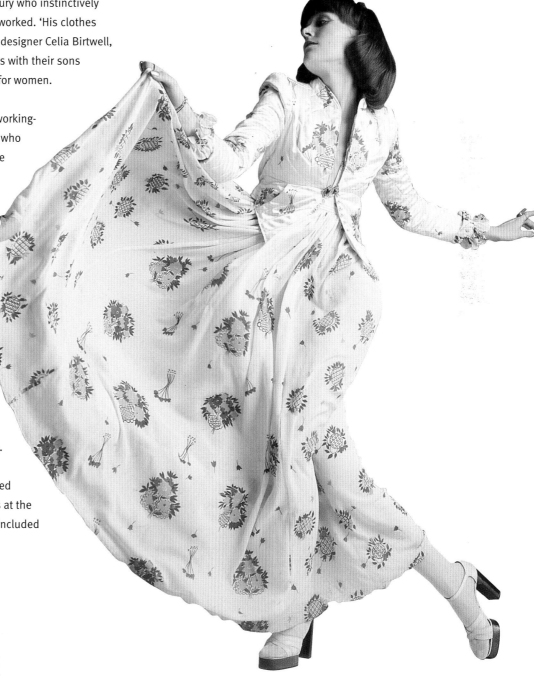

RIGHT **An eloquent collaboration with Ossie Clark on shape, Celia Birtwell on print. Circular white georgette dress and quilted satin jacket, 1973.**

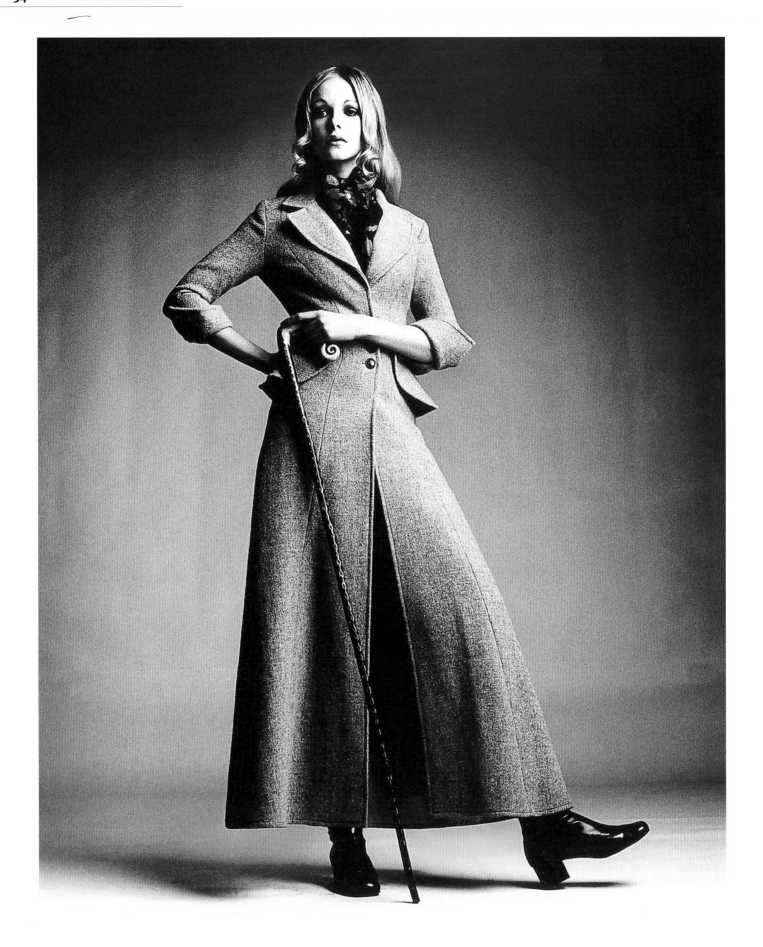

The 1970s were not easy for Clark: there were a series of comebacks, divorce from Celia in 1973 and legal wranglings in the bankruptcy courts. By the 1990s he had dropped out of the industry; he became a Buddhist and made occasional one-offs for private clients. Despite his premature demise, and tragic death at the age of 54, Clark's legacy of extraordinary dresses remains. 'I don't care how much anything costs as long as it's beautiful,' he told *The Sunday Times* in 1970. A heartfelt sentiment which characterizes many of the century's most brilliantly talented designers.

CLEMENTS RIBEIRO

Founded by Suzanne Clements and Inacia Ribeiro in 1993
Suzanne Clements, Born: Epsom, England, 1969
Inacia Ribeiro, Born: Itapecerica, Brazil, 1964

'Minimal dressing had become so uniform, we felt that romantic and feminine was the only way to go,' said Inacia Ribeiro, summing up his collection in 1997. The couple, who met while they were students at Central Saint Martins College of Art and Design in London, graduated with first-class honours in 1991 and married a year later. They worked as design consultants in Brazil before forming their own company in 1993. Clements Ribeiro are part of the new wave of British designers who mix colour, form and fabric in what they call an 'irreverent take on traditional elegance'. Their influences range from urban gypsies and faded opulence to Elizabethan tailoring and textures, and the colours of the sea.

CLERGERIE, Robert

Born: Paris, France, 1934

Clergerie shoes are synonymous with luxury, quality, and a constant attention to detail. They appeared in the film *Indecent Proposal* (1993) as part of the accoutrements of a millionaire's working wardrobe. Robert Clergerie is a fervent believer in simplicity: 'Black is practical. It continues,' he said in 1992. 'You mustn't confuse people with reality. It mixes them up.'

In 1992 he was awarded a design award from the Fashion Footwear Association of New York and opened a new store in Manhattan's SoHo. Father of three, fluent in English, and able to talk eloquently about the shape of shoes to come, Clergerie launched an exhibition of his life's work in Paris in March 1995, which travelled to New York and Hong Kong, and finished at the Shoe Museum in the shoemaking capital of Romans, France.

COLONNA, Jean

Born: Oran, Algeria, 1955

Jean Colonna learnt his craft at Balmain before launching his own label in 1985. It was not until fashion entered its deconstruction period in the early 1990s that Colonna found his métier. His look is simple without being dull, interesting yet not too extreme. Colonna is not precious about design: he regularly uses inexpensive fabrics and raw methods of finishing.

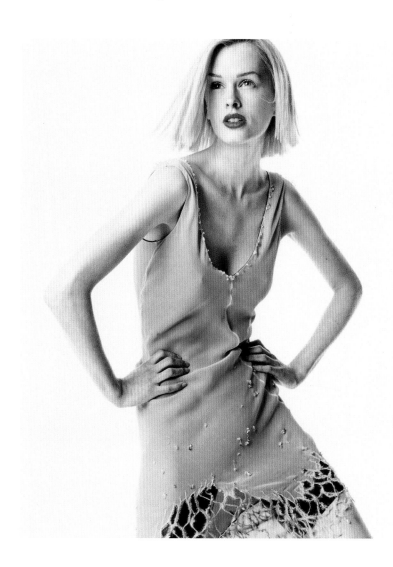

opposite Ossie Clark's 'last word in long coats', 1976: made from mist-pink Harris tweed, wasp-waisted, the silhouette stretched to the ankles.

right Elegantly distressed slip in silk chiffon, interspersed with diamanté pieces in Clements Ribeiro's 1998 'seabed' dress.

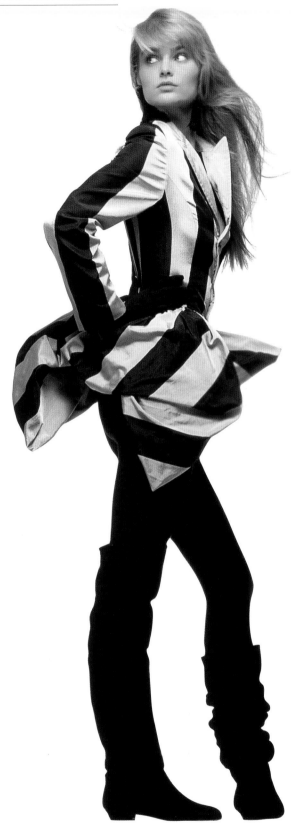

COMME DES GARÇONS

FOUNDED BY REI KAWAKUBO IN 1973
BORN: TOKYO, JAPAN, 1942

In 1981 there were four fashion capitals – Paris, London, Milan and New York – Tokyo was about to become the fifth. Comme des Garçons' mantra was monochrome colours, random elastication and a quest to turn conventional pattern cutting on its head. 'Red is Black' declared its founder, Rei Kawakubo. The shade, which for a century had been associated with mourning, was about to become the uniform of the fashionable.

Daughter of a university lecturer, Rei Kawakubo studied fine art at Keio University, Tokyo, and then went on to work for the advertising department of a chemical company. Disillusioned, she progressed to styling – an unusual occupation at the time. Comme des Garçons was established in 1973; two years later Kawakubo showed in Tokyo, and opened her first shop a year after that. But it was not until she showed in Paris in 1981 that the full force of the Japanese influence filtered through. What the audience saw was a shock to the system: random ruching, irregular hems, asymmetric seams and crinkled surfaces. *Vogue* called it 'oblique chic'.

Like her contemporaries, Issey Miyake and Yohji Yamamoto, Rei Kawakubo is an intellectual designer for whom fashion is a fine art. Her clothes require a different thought level, her pieces destroy pre-conceived ideas. The Comme des Garçons' concept sticks to the same principles: minimalist display and perplexing cuts. Often the uninitiated cannot understand where Kawakubo is coming from: sometimes shapeless and complicated, complex and baffling, a Comme des Garçons collection exposes the inner workings of a lapel, leaves edges unfinished and reduces a sweater to an unintelligible mass of boiled wool. In the autumn/winter 1996 collection, Kawakubo experimented with padded humps. The end product – nicknamed Quasimodo by the tabloid press for obvious reasons – had removable pads positioned in a variety of places. Her biannual magazine *Six* (from sixth sense), with its esoteric photographs and references to Zen, will probably one day be the subject of Freudian analysis.

Despite its unorthodox associations, Comme des Garçons has populist appeal: there are more than 300 outlets in 33 countries worldwide. Rei Kawakubo was the first to use 'real' people as catwalk models, including Hollywood stars Dennis Hopper, Matt Dillon, John Malkovich and John Hurt. Wearer of austere expressions and giver of few interviews, Kawakubo said, in *Rei Kawakubo and Comme des Garçons* (1990), 'What I do is concerned with the long term, and yet fashion is cyclical. It is a paradox, but it doesn't bother me. It's always exciting to do a new collection.'

ABOVE **Comme des Garçons' angular jacket of 1986 'with maverick swagged peplum', in Venetian striped polyester satin.**

OPPOSITE **A series of stripes, any which way but straight, highlight the complexity of cut in a Comme des Garçons suit, 1996.**

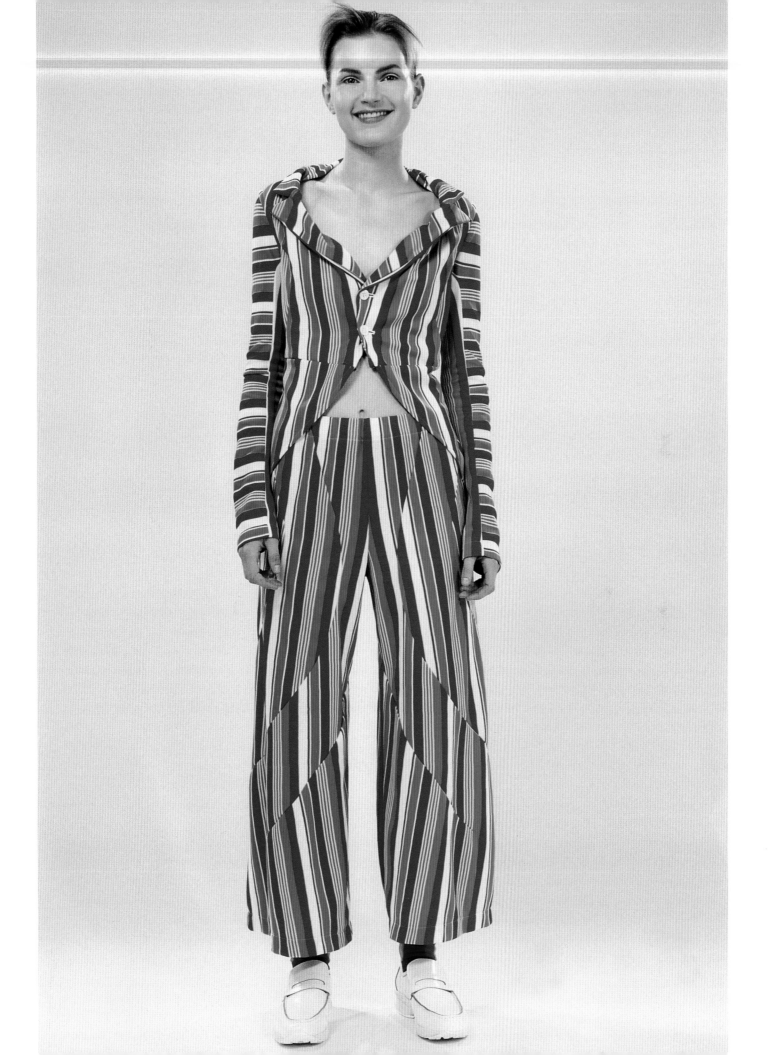

CONNOLLY, Sybil

BORN: SWANSEA, WALES, 1921
DIED: DUBLIN, IRELAND, 1998

When Dublin staged its first international dress show in the autumn of 1953 at Dunsany Castle, Sybil Connolly, the most famous name in Irish fashion, was the star. Born in Wales but with an Irish father, Connolly served an apprenticeship at Bradleys the dressmakers in 1938, where she attended fittings for the ailing Queen Mary, and moved to Dublin when she was 17 years old. A superb self-publicist, Connolly made it onto the cover of *Life*, dressed a series of aristocratic figures and became a friend of Jacqueline Kennedy. The Connolly style mixed American shapes and Irish content – simple linens, Donegal tweeds and Aran wool. When Jacqueline Kennedy visited Ireland in July 1967, she visited Connolly and wore one of her linen pieces in an official White House portrait.

Sybil Connolly established herself in a mansion in Merrion Square, Dublin, eventually paring down her business to cater only for a coterie of loyal clients, while writing books on Irish homes and gardens, and designing crystal and pottery for Tiffany & Co.

CONRAN, Jasper

BORN: LONDON, ENGLAND, 1959

Descended from a family of creatives and high achievers, Jasper Conran trained at Parson's School of Design in New York and then worked briefly at Fiorucci, Wallis and a clothing manufacturer in Barnsley, England. With the aid of a bank loan, he founded his own business in 1979, initially working from his father's Regent's Park house. In 1982 *Vogue* was calling Jasper Conran a 'British superlative'. At 26 years of age, he won the British Designer of the Year Award and had a turnover of £2.5 million. In 1991 he was nominated by *Tatler* as Mary Quant's tip for the top 'because he makes clothes women want to wear'.

Jasper Conran is one of the few designers who can switch from menswear to womenswear, from commercial, wearable clothes to watchable theatrical costumes. He rarely confuses the two. Conran has designed many times for the theatre including The Scottish Ballet's production of *Sleeping Beauty*, *My Fair Lady* directed by Simon Callow, and Jean Anouilh's *The Rehearsal*, for which he won a Laurence Olivier Award in 1990. His bridesmaids' dresses for the wedding of Lady Sarah Armstrong-Jones stand out as some of the most stunning ever produced.

COPPERWHEAT BLUNDELL

FOUNDED BY LEE COPPERWHEAT AND PAMELA BLUNDELL IN 1992

The Copperwheat Blundell partnership has a firm foundation built on solid experience from both sides. Lee Copperwheat studied tailoring at Tresham College in Northampton, at the London College of Fashion and at Aquascutum. Pamela Blundell trained at Southampton University, won the Smirnoff Best Young Designer fashion award in 1987, designed with John Flett and was commissioned to design a capsule collection for Liberty.

In 1997 Copperwheat Blundell launched CB OUTLINE, a collection which includes modern fabrics and has a sporty appeal. In the same year, they presented their first catwalk show in Japan. Their design experience is diverse, ranging from uniforms for Marco Pierre White's *Titanic* restaurant to clients including Cameron Diaz and The Corrs.

COURRÈGES, André

BORN: PAU, FRANCE, 1923

One of many designers of the 1960s who claims to have invented the mini, André Courrèges was mesmerized by space travel. In the years before the first man landed on the moon, Courrèges went crazy: silver trousers, moon boots, white plastic sunglasses – with slits echoing the shape of the eyelashes. The Courrèges look was clean, streamlined, and always looking to the future – white on white, silver on silver, sequins with moon boots, and space helmets accessorizing everything from shift dresses to trousersuits. Naturally, Andy Warhol was a fan.

Having originally trained as an air force pilot, Courrèges later enrolled at a training college for the clothing industry in Paris. In 1947 he worked as a designer at Jeanne Laufrie, and in 1951 for Cristobal Balenciaga. Balenciaga became Courrèges' mentor, making a loan available to enable him to set up a business with his partner Coqueline Barrière in 1961.

Courrèges showed his first mini in 1964, with *Vogue* declaring his version the shortest in Paris. Shortly afterwards, he announced that his designs were being plagiarized and suspended giving shows until 1967, but continued to design for private customers. In 1968 Courrèges built his own futuristic factory in Pau – a suitably semi-transparent structure with glass

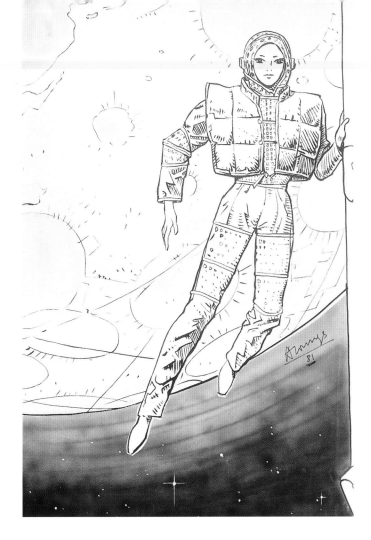

LEFT **Courrèges' view of fashion in the year 2000: 'she is constantly ascending, she's tied to the cosmos, hence, her spacesuit'.**

CRAHAY, Jules-François

BORN: LIÈGE, BELGIUM, 1917
DIED: MONTE CARLO, MONACO, 1988

Son of a couturière, Jules-François Crahay began his career early. At 13 years old he was already working as an illustrator at his mother's couture house. In 1934 Crahay moved to Paris to study couture and then returned to join his mother's establishment, where he helped dress Belgium's high society for two years. During the Second World War he was captured and imprisoned for four years. Crahay then joined Nina Ricci – his 1959 collection was rapturously received – and defected to Jeanne Lanvin in 1963, succeeding Antonio del Castillo and directing the collections for 20 years. 'I have no use for afternoon clothes,' he once remarked, 'fashion leaps from the little morning suit to the evening gown.'

CREED, Charles Southey

BORN: PARIS, FRANCE, 1909
DIED: LONDON, ENGLAND, 1966

Son of Henry Creed of Paris – who claimed to be the first tailor to introduce tweeds into women's suits – Charles Creed was one of the movers and shakers of British fashion in the 1940s. 'He was pre-destined to design exquisite clothes,' said *Vogue* in 1946. 'Like any artist he seeks perfection, in his case it is tailored perfection.'

Educated in France, England and Germany, Creed joined his father's business – established by his ancestors in 1710 – before settling in London. At 17 years old, he travelled to Vienna to study tailoring and design. In 1941 he produced utility designs and, after the Second World War, opened his own London house. He married Patricia Cunningham, a fashion editor at *Vogue*, in 1948.

Charles Creed was in possession of one of the finest collections of lead soldiers and porcelains of the Napoleonic era. In his autobiography, *Maid to Measure* (1961), he claims to have invented the concept of boutiques in 1939 and concludes, 'I have grown older and grey and rather bald in the pursuit of my profession and the opposite sex – and I still cannot think of a better way to spend one's time.'

walls. Two collections were produced by Jean-Charles de Castelbajac in 1994. Still looking to the future, in 1997 André Courrèges launched his perfume 2020.

COX, Patrick

BORN: EDMONTON, ALBERTA, CANADA, 1963

Most famous for his Wannabe loafer, which enjoyed phenomenal success in the early 1990s, Patrick Cox has now changed tack from concentrating solely on shoes to accessories and clothing.

Cox emigrated from Canada to England in 1983 to attend Cordwainers College, London – the only establishment to specialize specifically in shoe design. While still a student, he worked with Vivienne Westwood on her autumn/winter 1984 collection. In 1985 Cox set up his own company – which commissions for British designers including John Galliano – where he continued for six seasons. Since then, he has produced collections for Anna Sui, Katharine Hamnett and, in 1990, Lanvin's prêt-à-porter collection. In 1991 Patrick Cox opened his first shop in London, selling antiques alongside his bestselling loafer.

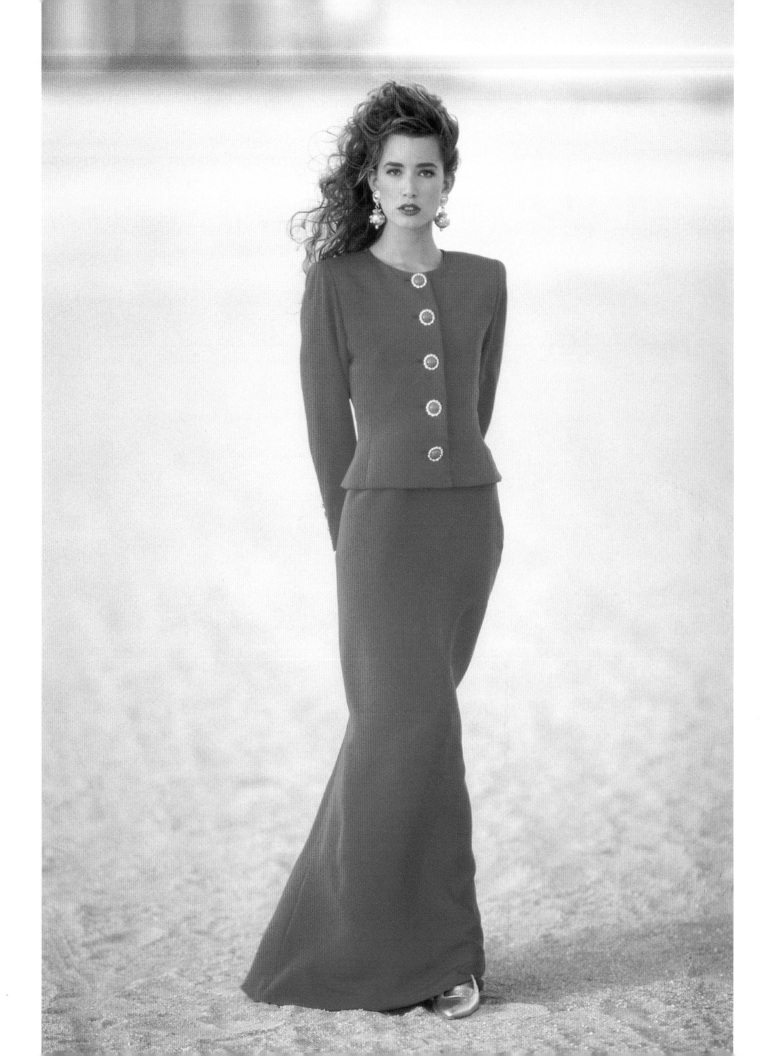

DACHÉ, Lilly

BORN: BÉGLES, FRANCE, 1907
DIED: LOUVECIENNES, FRANCE, 1989

The personification of the American Dream, Lilly Daché was a French immigrant who, within the space of a decade, became an enduring household name for chic millinery.

Having learnt her craft at Reboux in Paris, Daché defected to New York in 1924, becoming a millinery sales assistant at Macy's department store. She then worked at The Bonnet Shop, before buying the business and opening additional outlets in Chicago and Florida. At the height of her fame, Daché was collaborating with Hollywood costume designer Travis Banton. Her speciality, turbans draped directly onto the head, enabled her to swathe fabric around some of Tinsel Town's starriest crowns, including Carole Lombard, Betty Grable, Lorette Young and Marlene Dietrich. Daché was also famous for close-fitting, brimmed cloche hats, snoods and caps. Her autobiography, *Talking Through My Hats*, was published in 1946; in the late 1950s, she employed Halston as an assistant.

DE LA RENTA, Oscar

BORN: SANTO DOMINGO, DOMINICAN REPUBLIC, 1932

Colourful and sociable, Oscar de la Renta studied art in Spain, worked for Cristobal Balenciaga and was then employed as an assistant to Antonio del Castillo at Lanvin. He cites Coco Chanel and Balenciaga as the major talents of the century.

In 1967 de la Renta married the editor-in-chief of French *Vogue*, Françoise de la Languade. He later married New York socialite, Annette Reed, in 1989. De la Renta lives in Connecticut, but also owns an opulent apartment in New York and a luxurious retreat in La Romana in the Dominican Republic. Famous for his opulent eveningwear, which is both vibrant and tasteful, his clients list is a roll call of America's socially significant – Liza Minelli, Nancy Reagan, Joan Collins, Ivana Trump, Jacqueline Onassis and Fay Dunaway – and his friends include Dr Henry Kissinger and television presenter Barbara Walters.

OPPOSITE **Oscar de la Renta on top form: fitted sunset-orange jacket in silk crepe with gilt-edged buttons, over a matching full-skirted dress, 1989.**

De la Renta is well known for his services to charity: he set up a children's home, Casa de Niños, in his native Dominican Republic – and adopted one of their children, Moises, at 8 months old.

Although de la Renta's signature is flamboyance and colour, he has survived major swings in fashion. In 1991, at 58 years of age and with annual sales of $350 million, de la Renta showed his collection for the first time in an attempt to broaden his client base – it was also the first time an American designer had shown in Paris. The public relations exercise paid off: two years later, in 1993, he was appointed designer to Pierre Balmain – making him the first American designer to head a Parisian couture house. His career had, at last, come full circle.

DE LISI, Ben

BORN: BROOKLYN, NEW YORK, USA, 1955

Winner of British Fashion's Glamour Award two years running, Ben de Lisi was born in Brooklyn, raised in Long Island and graduated from the Pratt Institute, New York, in 1977. He worked briefly for Bloomingdales while he was still at college, designed a range of T-shirts which he sold to Saks Fifth Avenue, and spent four years with a young designer called Penelope before launching his own menswear line called 'Benedetto' – his full Christian name.

In 1982 de Lisi opened a French restaurant, Ciboure, in London's Belgravia. He designed a capsule collection of ten pieces using job lot fabric – cut on tables above the restaurant – and made them up himself between sittings. He pounded the pavement and ended up with £30,000 worth of orders. De Lisi excels at swimwear and eveningwear – in December 1998 he opened his first shop in Belgravia's Elizabeth Street.

DE PRÉMONVILLE, Myrène

BORN: HENDAYE, FRANCE, 1949

Known for her use of colour and fastidious tailoring with a slight theatrical bent, Myrène De Prémonville was described by *Vogue* in 1987 as 'the new discovery of the past two seasons ... her collection neither based on a lifestyle, nor a customer, but the creative urge of someone who has worked half her life in fashion.'

Working exclusively with French fabrics and French manufacturers, De Prémonville's clothes – including dresses for day and evening, and knits – blend a youthful spirit of innovation with conservative Gallic chic.

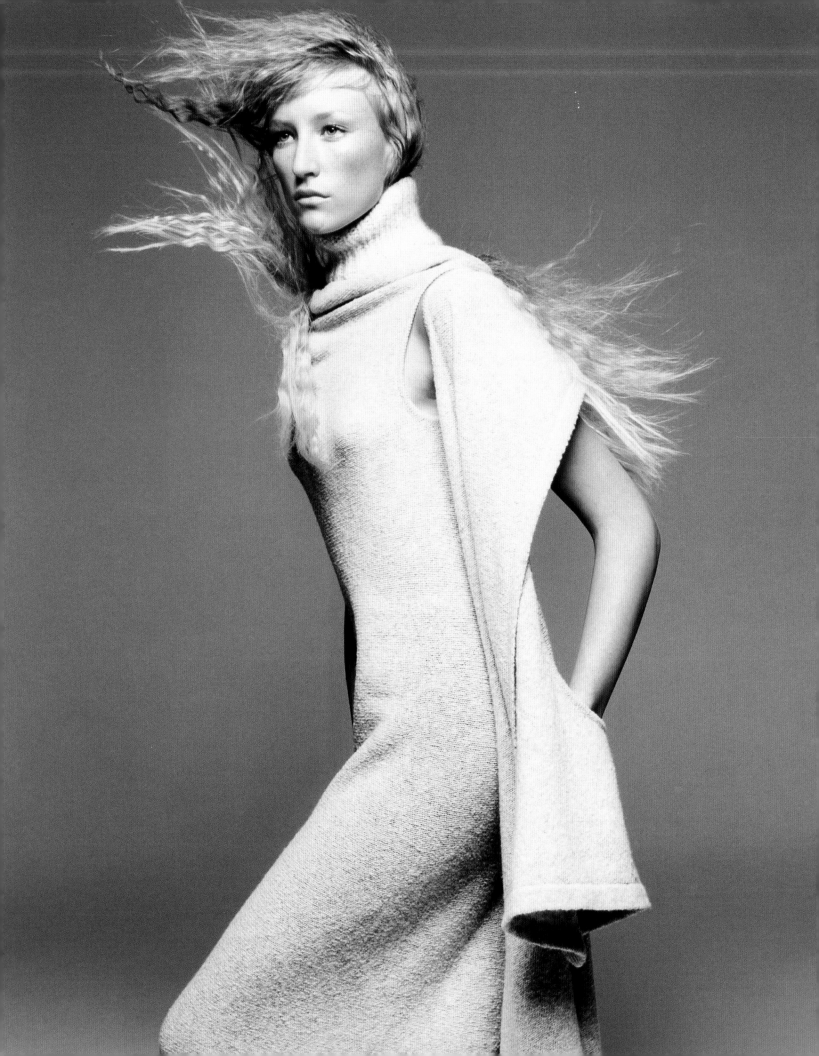

DELAUNAY, Sonia

BORN: ODESSA, UKRAINE, 1885
DIED: PARIS, FRANCE, 1979

Painter, textile designer and supreme colourist, Sonia Delaunay's dresses epitomize the meaning of modernity. Abstract and angular, her designs contain the juxtaposition of geometric shapes and squares and developed out of Cubism. Delaunay's designs were worn by Nancy Cunard, Gloria Swanson and a host of French film stars and international artists. She delivered a lecture at the Sorbonne in Paris in 1926 called 'The Influence of Painting on Fashion Design'. An amazing 94 years old when she died, Delaunay left a rich seam of work and dresses, which look as if they were designed yesterday.

DEMEULEMEESTER, Ann

BORN: KORTRIJK, BELGIUM, 1959

Ann Demeulemeester is a member of a group of experimental designers who emerged from Belgium in the mid-1980s. Termed deconstructivists, they achieved recognition by creating raw, elemental, non-traditional clothes. Demeulemeester designs with a close attention to detail and prefers to concentrate on pairing unusual fabrics, rather than focusing on colour and ornament. Although she is a meticulous planner, her clothes always look uncontrived. Her style is a melting pot of punk, gothic and Japanese; long coats and dresses in draped fabrics have become her signature, together with halter-neck vests and trousers and skirts which expose the hip bone. Often contradictory, Demeulemeester combines unconventional cutting and tailoring with distressed fabrics and crucifixes, and always mixes the austere with the avant-garde.

Demeulemeester studied fashion design at the Royal Academy of Fine Arts in Antwerp and worked freelance before launching her own line in 1985. She showed her first collection in a Parisian art gallery and opened her Paris showroom in 1992. In 1996 she produced her first menswear line. Her celebrity clients include Madonna and Courtney Love.

OPPOSITE **Demeulemeester deconstructs the knit: a cream merino wool cape dress with detachable polo neck collar, 1998.**

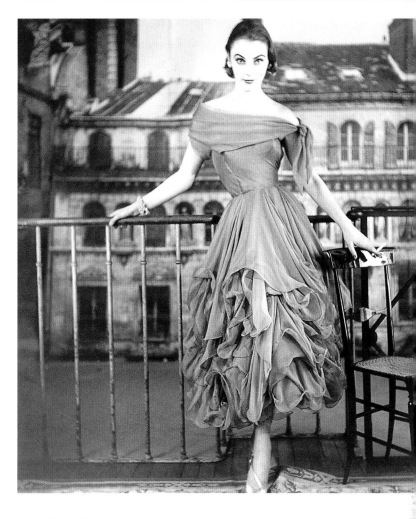

ABOVE **Flounced, smoky mauve skirt, caught up unevenly in tiers like curls of smoke on one of Dessès's many chiffon dresses, 1953.**

DESSÈS, Jean

BORN: ALEXANDRIA, EGYPT, 1904
DIED: ATHENS, GREECE, 1970

In 1950 *Vogue* described Jean Dessès, an Egyptian-born Greek, as daring and influential. 'Dessès creates with a hand that is dashing and unafraid. The inspired results: flattering décolletages; clothes with easy and young movement of line.' A couturier who came to prominence in post-war Paris, Dessès had become so famous by the turn of the 1950s that he created the 'Jean Dessès American Collection', a range that was designed and sold directly through wholesalers. He was acclaimed as one of *Vogue*'s 'Names in the News', 'hailed and applauded by American store buyers, recognised and respected by your customers.'

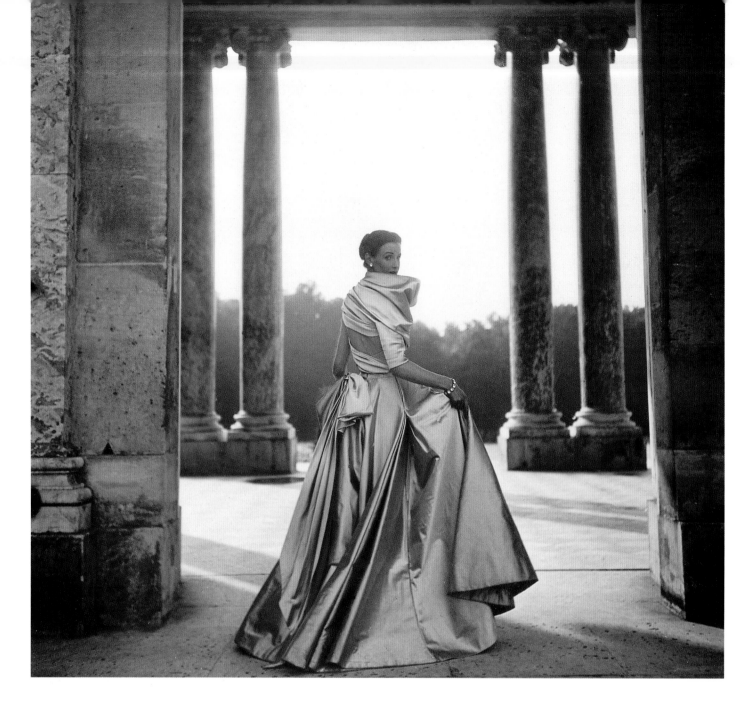

DIOR, Christian

BORN: GRANVILLE, FRANCE, 1905
DIED: MONTECATINI, ITALY, 1957

Christian Dior was responsible for the pivotal point in twentieth-century fashion. His New Look shook the world, brought women back to life and became fashion's most powerful political statement. Dior studied political science at École des Sciences Politiques in Paris from 1920–25. He served in the French army and worked as an art dealer, illustrator and designer at Piguet and Lelong before launching his curvaceous controversy on an unsuspecting world in December 1946. Heralded an overnight sensation, Dior was, in fact, 41 years old.

Dior's New Look was equal parts fashion and social revolution. It was a female seducer with explosive elements: excessive fabric in a period of austerity; a return to femininity after wartime suppression; a taste of glamour after years of drab. Although sketches smuggled out of Paris during the war were predicting a return to undulation, it was Dior who delivered. 'The prime need of fashion is to please and attract,' he mused in his memoirs, *Dior by Dior* (1957). 'Uniformity is the mother of boredom.'

Dior – whose preferred places for sketching were the bed or bath – dominated *Vogue*'s collection reports for a decade. 'His ideas were fresh and put over with great authority,' wrote *Vogue* in 1947. 'His clothes were beautifully made, essentially Parisian, deeply feminine …' Like Balenciaga, Dior's prime concern was silhouette and form, and he admitted that he could happily produce all of his collections in black or white. 'Colour cannot transform a failure of a dress into a success,' he said. 'It merely plays a supporting role in a cast where the cut is the star performer.'

Dior's preoccupation was the formulation of new lines: the Oblique line of 1950, the Oval line in spring 1951, the Envol in autumn, the Princess line, the Profile line in 1952, the H line in 1954, the A line followed by the Y line in 1955. Although the collections generated valuable publicity, and spawned countless imitations, it was the lucrative contracts with licensees that culminated in sales of over £700 million. In one season alone, 2,500 customers passed through the Christian Dior salons.

The house which Dior built continued after his death. The legend was intact. Yves Saint Laurent, who had joined Dior as design assistant in 1955 – the only person to be given this unique position – was appointed chief designer at the tender age of 21. His first collection, the Trapeze line in 1958, was a radical departure. Two years later, when Saint Laurent was conscripted into the French army and suffered a nervous breakdown, he passed the baton to Marc Bohan, who remained there for 28 years.

A major retrospective celebrating the house of Dior was held at the Musée des Arts de la Mode, Paris, in 1987. In 1989 Italian Gianfranco Ferre succeeded Marc Bohan and, finally, John Galliano – the first British designer to head an established Parisian house – moved from Givenchy and replaced Ferre in 1996, declaring Dior 'the punk of his time'.

OPPOSITE **Christian Dior's 'intricately beautiful' evening gown of 1948 in pearl grey satin with asymmetric wrapped neckline and a single sleeve.**

RIGHT **Dior under the direction of brilliant maverick John Galliano: long, sparkling dress of antique silver paillettes, 1999.**

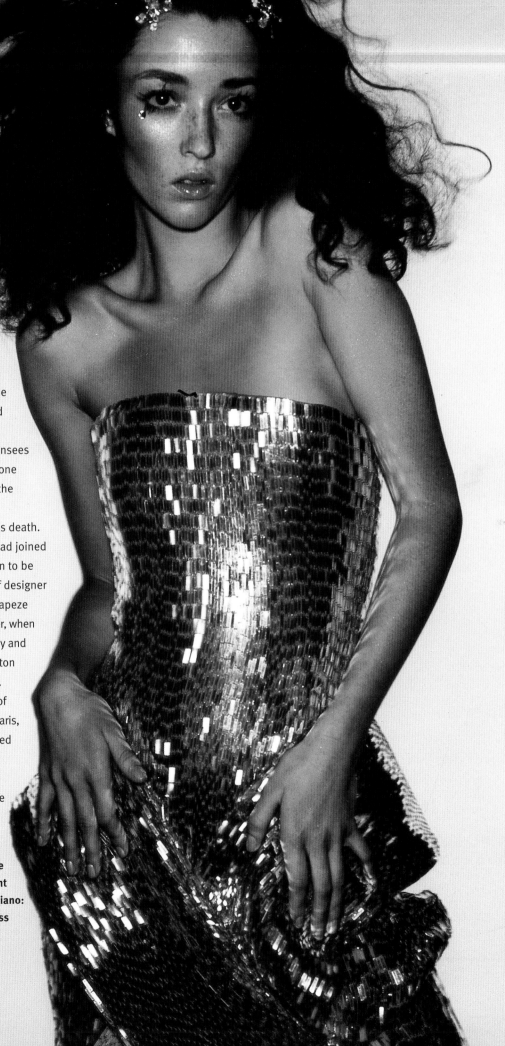

DŒUILLET, House of

FOUNDED BY GEORGES DŒUILLET IN 1900

One of the most-featured labels in *Vogue*'s early years, the house of Dœuillet was known for its attention to detail, rather than for directional design.

Having worked as a manager at Callot Sœurs – who specialized in fine lace and delicate touches – Georges Dœuillet branched out on his own. He situated his house in one of the royal mansions on the place Vendôme in Paris, where he forged a reputation for exquisite eveningwear. In 1914 he was made president of the French Syndicate of Dressmakers and was described in *Vogue* as 'not pronounced in his personality, but his wonderful head for business and his saneness make him a bulwark for many of the other couturiers'. In 1929 Dœuillet merged with the house of Doucet.

DOLCE & GABBANA

FOUNDED BY DOMENICO DOLCE AND STEFANO GABBANA IN 1985

Dolce & Gabbana put sex into Sicily. They swept away the preconceived ideas of widows and vendettas and reinvented it with seduction and shades of Sophia Loren. Dolce & Gabbana are experts in mixed metaphors of flyaway beading, corsetry and cleavage, often accessorized by curled locks and a sweep of 1950s-style eyeliner. Launched in 1985, their early collections concentrated on corsetry, the promotion of cotton/Lycra underwear as outerwear. In 1993 the duo designed costumes for Madonna's Girlie Show. By 1997 they were Hollywood hotshots, dressing the stars for a variety of awards. 'The show is only fantasy,' said Stefano, underplaying their reputation in 1997, 'it's not even that representative of what we do. People think Dolce: glamour, curves, sexy. But we also do suits, cardigans, skirts – clothes women can wear to work.'

DOUCET, Jacques

BORN: PARIS, FRANCE, 1853
DIED: PARIS, FRANCE, 1929

'Next to Poiret, Doucet is the most amazing personality among the men in the dressmaking world of Paris,' commented *Vogue* in 1914. 'He is often called the most elegant man in Paris.' The celebrated house of Doucet was established in 1816 by the

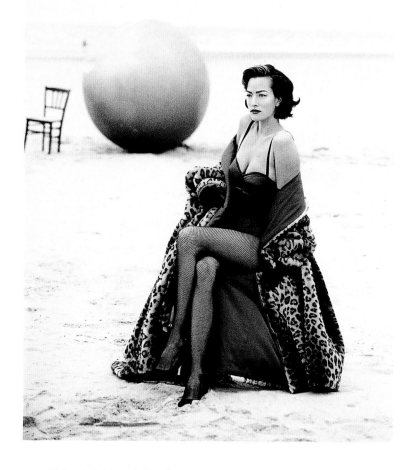

ABOVE **Dolce & Gabbana's 'movie star glamour' of 1991: fake leopardskin coat with deep shawl collar; scarlet silk corset with black stitching.**

grandmother of Jacques Doucet. The building – a house already renowned for making fine lingerie – was situated on boulevard Saint-Martin. Maison Doucet later relocated to rue de la Paix. In 1877 it began making gowns and costumes.

Jacques Doucet was a patron of the arts, an authority on French eighteenth-century history, with an instinct for the grand occasion – he collaborated on countless theatrical productions, owned a hotel and, it is said, invested six million francs in rare books. *Vogue* assessed his collections as embodying 'a gracious elegance and a fineness of workmanship which could not be surpassed'. In 1932, after a merger with Dœuillet, the house closed.

DUFF GORDON, Lucile

BORN: LONDON, ENGLAND, 1862

DIED: LONDON, ENGLAND, 1935

A single mother in an era when divorce was associated with disgrace, Lucile Duff Gordon had a colourful personal life, a high profile and a 21-inch waist in 1899. Married at 18, she was divorced by her mid-twenties with a 5-year-old daughter, Esme. In 1900 she met and married Sir Cosmo Duff Gordon, whose social connections invariably helped her client list.

Lucile, as she was known, advocated the elimination of the corset, a return to Grecian lines, and put colour into hair years before punk. Although Paul Poiret pioneered the new silhouette, Lucile promoted the Empire line. She broke into the American market, made theatrical designs and met Emmeline Pankhurst when she was advocating votes for women. Sister to novelist Elinor Glyn and pioneer of her time, Lady Duff Gordon came to the conclusion that women should be seen but not heard. In her autobiography, *Discretions and Indiscretions*, published in 1932, she writes, 'I do not think that, on the whole, it is good for a woman with a temperament. It is much better for her to be a vegetable, and certainly much safer, but I never had a choice.'

RIGHT AND BELOW **Lucile's 'exotic, Oriental frocks' of 1917 reveal bare flesh, ankles, arms, a flash of cleavage and gold lace trousers.**

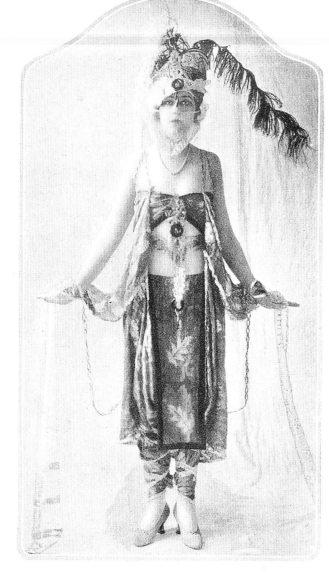

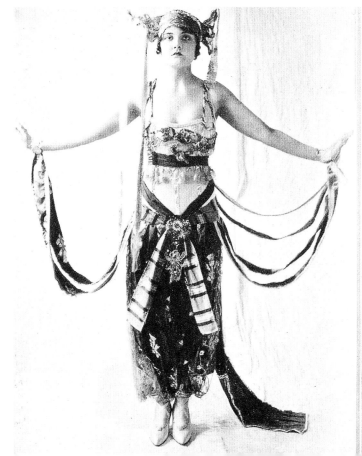

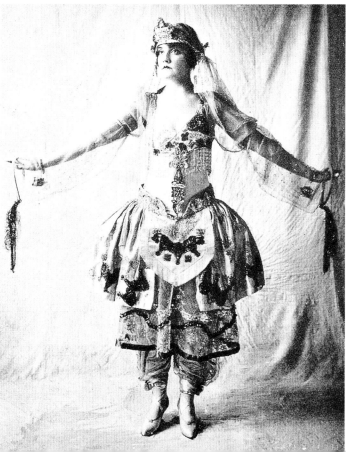

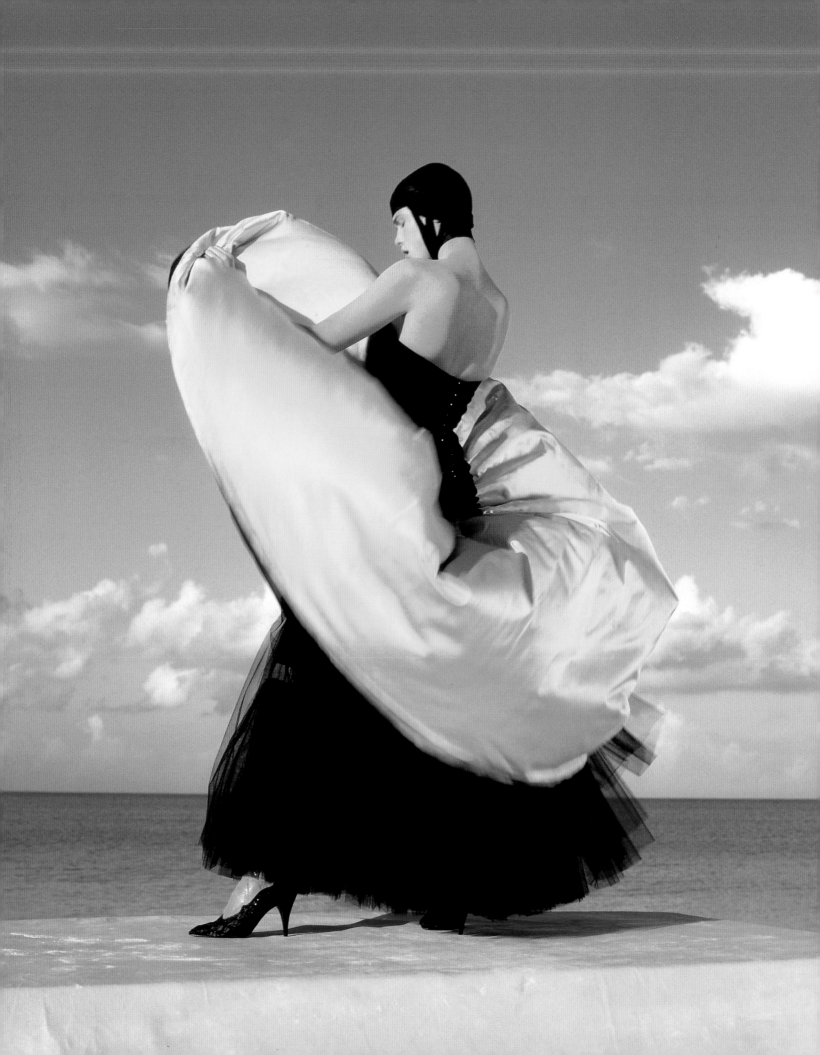

EDELSTEIN, Victor

BORN: LONDON, ENGLAND, 1947

'She likes body-conscious clothes, and why not? She's got a fabulous figure,' said British couturier Victor Edelstein of his most famous client in 1987. Edelstein will forever be associated with the bare-shouldered velvet dress he made for Diana, Princess of Wales, which she wore while dancing with John Travolta at President Reagan's White House State Dinner in 1985. At the Christie's auction in 1997 it eclipsed every other gown, selling at the record price of $222,500.

Descended from a line of dressmakers – both his father and grandfather were in the business – Edelstein trained at Alexon and a Paris couture boutique. In 1967, after several dismissals for being too dreamy, he worked for Barbara Hulanicki at Biba for three years. After a period of self-employment, he became assistant designer at the London couture branch of Christian Dior. He married art dealer Annamaria in 1973 and started his own ready-to-wear business in 1978. In 1982 he decided to concentrate solely on couture.

At 46 years old, Edelstein hung up his scissors and decided to retire. His reasons were both financial and psychological: as he told the *Evening Standard* in 1993, 'I've spent eleven years being polite and constantly watching what I say. I look at something that's tight and instead of saying "We'll let that out", I have to say "We'll ease that over the hips."' Currently painting landscapes in Venice, treading on eggshells is no longer one of his concerns.

ELBAZ, Alber

BORN: CASABLANCA, MOROCCO, 1961

The first designer to direct Yves Saint Laurent's Rive Gauche line, Alber Elbaz is an Israeli-American with a fantastic sense of proportion and healthy sense of humour. Elbaz trained with America's foremost minimalist, Geoffrey Beene, for seven years before being offered an opportunity he couldn't refuse. He first designed at Guy Laroche and presented his first collection at the Carrousel du Louvre in Paris on 13 March 1991. On 2 November 1998 Alber Elbaz joined Yves Saint Laurent as artistic director for women's ready to wear, presenting his last collection for Rive Gauche in Spring 2000.

OPPOSITE **Victor Edelstein's wild side: silk grosgrain bustier and golden yellow duchesse satin skirt over a black tulle petticoat, 1986.**

ELLIS, Perry

BORN: PORTSMOUTH, VIRGINIA, USA, 1940
DIED: NEW YORK, NEW YORK, USA, 1986

Perry Ellis designed sportswear in the true sense of the word. Clean lines, crisp fabrics – clothes that crossed the border between lounging and activity. Ellis knew all about the ins and outs of sportswear, having started his career as a sportswear buyer for Miller & Rhoads, a Virginian department store, later taking up a position of designer. He had degrees in both business and retailing, and his diverse experience culminated in an astute understanding of commercial design.

Ellis formed his own label, Perry Ellis International, in 1978. His easy-to-wear slouch look – consisting of loose trousers, layered tunics and oversized sweaters – became his signature menswear and sportswear line in conjunction with Levi Strauss. Elected president of the Council of Fashion Designers of America in 1984, he said, 'My clothes are friendly – like people you've known for a long time, but who continue to surprise you. Clothes must do the same.'

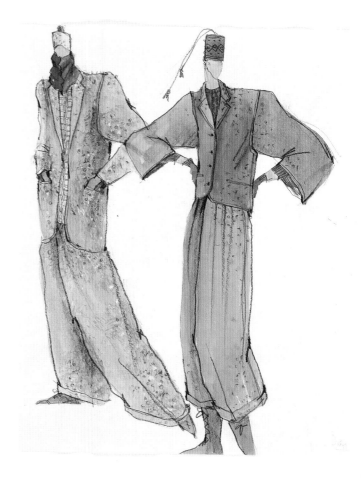

RIGHT **Loose tailoring, long lines and 'Chaplin bags' in Perry Ellis's Burren tweed suits, here drawn by Ellis himself.**

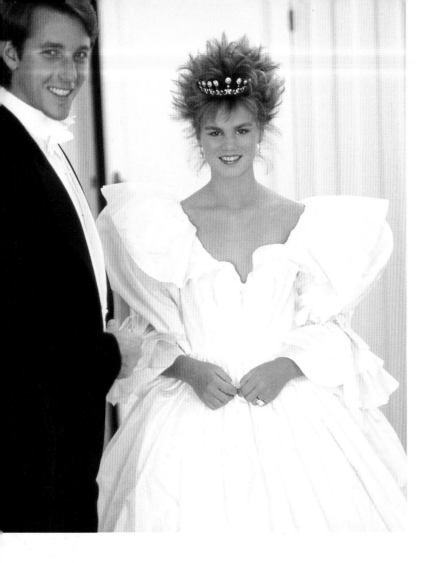

ENGLISH ECCENTRICS

FOUNDED BY HELEN DAVID IN 1983

Having trained at London's Camberwell School of Art and Central Saint Martins College of Art and Design, Helen David – founder of English Eccentrics – is known for her print, colour and quirky textiles, which mix the baroque with aesthetically pleasing shapes. Not limited to accessories, the English Eccentrics label also encompasses shirts, often with a Pucci-esque feel.

ESTRADA, Angel

BORN: BARCELONA, SPAIN, 1957
DIED: NEW YORK, NEW YORK, USA, 1989

A talented designer, who had a flair for combining sculptural shapes with fluid effects, Angel Estrada secured a *Vogue* front cover – a satin bustier with luggage zip – within his first year of business in November 1986.

Estrada's family relocated from Spain to New York when he was 3 years old. After studying briefly at Parson's School of Design, New York, he worked as a hair and make-up artist and then, in 1985, formed his own label, which he kept afloat without outside finance. After Estrada's death at the age of 31, the business was taken over by his sister Virginia, an artist and sculptor, who had collaborated with her brother on his collections.

EMANUEL,
David and Elizabeth

DAVID EMANUEL, BORN: BRIDGEND, WALES, 1952
ELIZABETH WEINER, BORN: LONDON, ENGLAND, 1953

The couple who have now gone their separate ways will forever be remembered as the designers behind the wedding dress of Diana, Princess of Wales. Unveiled on 31 July 1981, the most important royal wedding dress of the decade was made from pure silk taffeta overlaid with lace, mother-of-pearl sequins and pearls, with a double-flounce collar and 7.6-metre (25-foot) detachable train. A matching pochette and an umbrella were designed in the event of rain.

Already married when they entered the Royal College of Art in London, the Emanuels graduated in 1978 and launched their Mayfair boutique. They perfectly captured the mood of the moment – a mix of New Romantics and royal wedding fever. The then Lady Diana Spencer wore an Emanuel blouse for her first sitting for British *Vogue*. The Emanuels have since concentrated on their individual careers.

ETTEDGUI, Joseph

BORN: CASABLANCA, MOROCCO, 1936

Son of a French-Moroccan furniture retailer, Joseph Ettedgui emigrated to London in the late 1950s and trained to be a hairdresser. During the 1960s he began travelling to Paris to see the ready-to-wear collections. There, he met Kenzo, whose brightly-coloured sweaters he started to sell in the reception area of his King's Road salon. Before long, the clothes had eclipsed the hairdressing, and Joseph's first shop was established below the salon in the early 1970s.

Joseph has continued his winning-formula own label alongside international names – from Azzedine Alaïa to Helmut Lang, with John Galliano, Katharine Hamnett and a host of others in-between. In 1993 he moved into menswear, then furniture design and cafes – Joe's and L'Express – and one restaurant, Joe's Cafe. His shops, designed by architects Eva Jiricna and David Chipperfield, are appropriately modernistic – using steel, white and concrete colours as a background for the collections. He also has branches in Paris, Cannes and New York. As he told the *Observer* in 1987, 'Once a place becomes a meeting point, you get the business.'

FARHI, Nicole

BORN: NICE, FRANCE, 1946

Unpretentious clothes with nothing to prove are at the core of Nicole Farhi's philosophy. After studying fashion in Paris, Farhi freelanced at Agnès B and Jean-Charles de Castelbajac. She moved to Britain in 1973 and worked for French Connection with Stephen Marks. A decade later she formed her own label, and launched a menswear collection in 1989. Her flagship store on London's Sloane Street opened in October 1998. Like Joseph, she has expanded her business to include a restaurant – in her case Nicole's – situated beneath her Bond Street store. Farhi opened her first New York branch in 1999.

FATH, Jacques

BORN: LAFITTE, FRANCE, 1912
DIED: PARIS, FRANCE, 1954

Jacques Fath was the darling of the Parisian social scene, his name spoken in the same sentence as Cristobal Balenciaga and Christian Dior. Fath's style, however, was less breathtaking and more a celebration of the female form. Described by *Vogue* in the 1950s as 'a comet', Fath shot to fame after the Second World War, in the wake of the fashion revolution caused by Dior's New Look: women dressed according to the Paris directive and the press were, once again, frequenting the front row.

Fath had dressmaking in his blood – his great-grandmother was dressmaker to Empress Eugénie – but he started his career as a book-keeper. He showed his first collection in 1937, but it was in the post-war era of renewed optimism and femininity that he made his mark. While Balenciaga and Dior concentrated on sculpture and the invention of new proportions, Fath focused on undulating lines and elegant juxtaposition of colours.

'Persian lamb is dyed blue to trim a blue suit,' said *Vogue* in its collection report of September 1956. 'Fath carries the idea still further with green, red and purple.' During his short, sharp career, Fath made a lasting impression. A retrospective of his work was held in Paris in 1993.

FENDI

FOUNDED BY ADELE CASAGRANDE IN 1918

One of the largest and most important of the Italian fashion dynasties, Fendi began as a leather and fur workshop over a century ago. Its founder, Adele Casagrande, who married Eduardo Fendi in 1925, changed the company's name after the death of her father in 1954.

Although Fendi is inextricably linked with fur, the label is also known for its other lines – namely ready to wear and accessories. During the 30 years that Karl Lagerfeld has been associated with Fendi – he has designed their collections since 1965 – he has redirected the label from an anonymous luxury brand into a high-profile house with elitist connotations. Like the unmistakable Chanel logo, Fendi's logo is world-famous.

Over the past century fur has fallen in and out of favour with alarming regularity. Despite shifting tastes and phases of political correctness, Fendi has remained immovable, although customers in the late 1990s showed more interest in Fendi's chic accessories – the baguette bag was a phenomenal bestseller – than in making huge investments buying fur.

FÉRAUD, Louis

BORN: ARLES, FRANCE, 1921

Chic suits and sophisticated French tailoring are the signatures of Louis Féraud. Glamorous and wearable, his clothes appeal to groomed thirtysomethings and women of a 'certain age': his clothes were worn by Joan Collins during her *Dynasty* and *Dallas* periods, but have also been worn by Brigitte Bardot, Catherine Deneuve and Kim Novak.

Féraud served as a lieutenant in the French Resistance, and opened his first couture boutique in Cannes in 1955, which was patronized by movie stars. He became a costume designer before moving to Paris 20 years later. In 1984 he won the coveted Golden Thimble Award. An accomplished artist with a sensitive palette, he has held many exhibitions and is also an author – *L'Été du Pingouin* was published in 1975.

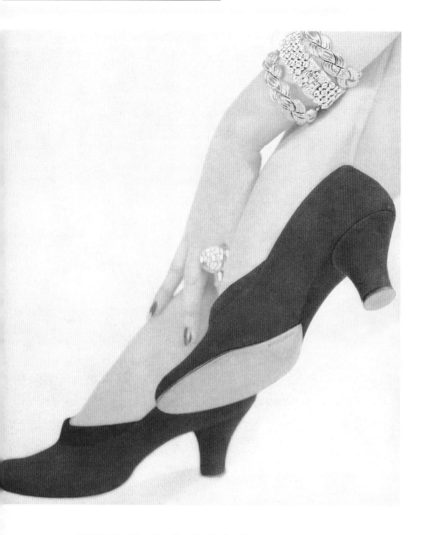

LEFT **The perfectly proportioned shoe from Ferragamo, featuring his gloved suede arch of 1952: 'it's all new, the colour, the shape, the spool heel.'**

FERRE, Gianfranco

BORN: LEGNANO, ITALY, 1944

Famously compared with Frank Lloyd Wright, Gianfranco Ferre has a rotund physique and aesthetic sensibility. His grandfather designed bicycles and his father was the owner of two factories. Ferre originally trained as an architect at Milan Polytechnic, graduating in 1969. His favourite architectural triumphs include the Institut du Monde Arabe in Paris and the Torre Velasca in Milan. Ferre's first official show was presented in a restaurant in Via San Murillo, Milan, in 1974. Four years later came his first collection, 'Gianfranco Ferre Donna', followed by a menswear line in 1982.

A doer rather than a talker, since 1983 Ferre has been a professor at the Domus Academy in Milan and financed the restoration of sixteenth-century frescoes. His intellectual approach and sensitivity to form and outline produces powerful designs – such as his voluminous organza shirts – as well as immaculate tailoring. In 1989, Ferre was appointed artistic director at Christian Dior, and his first collection – which he was told he had nine weeks to complete – occurred in the same year. With Grace Jones and Princess Michael of Kent in the front row, Ferre's first show for Dior was dedicated to Cecil Beaton's Ascot scene in *My Fair Lady* (1964), and featured Ferre's speciality – huge bows. It was described by *Vogue* as 'a matter of Dior discipline and Ferre flourish'. He was awarded Paris fashion's highest accolade, the Golden Thimble, on the final day of the collections.

Ferre continued with his own collection, and his career after leaving Dior in 1996 has included diffusion lines Ferre Sport, Ferre Jeans, Ferre Studio and Studio 000.1, as well as an experimental line, GIEFFEFFE.

FERRAGAMO, Salvatore

BORN: BONITO, ITALY, 1898
DIED: FIUMETTO, ITALY, 1960

Salvatore Ferragamo's supremacy in making innovative shoe shapes was a product of his apprenticeship with a craftsman in his native Italy. In 1923 he emigrated to America and opened a shoe shop in Santa Barbara, California, making couture shoes. His client list included Audrey Hepburn, Sophia Loren, the Duchess of Windsor and Eva Perón. He also worked with producer and director Cecil B De Mille. Ferragamo was a perfectionist and innovator. He worked with unusual materials – Cellophane, raffia, lace and crystal, as well as fish skin and sea leopard – and instigated new shapes, including the platform shoe, an ancient Chinese idea which he relaunched in 1938. Between 1927 and 1960 he produced 20,000 designs, and published his biography, *Shoemaker of Dreams* in 1957. He didn't care that his style was relentlessly plagiarized – Ferragamo was the original: 'Elegance and comfort are not incompatible, and whoever maintains the contrary simply doesn't know what he is talking about.'

OPPOSITE **Gianfranco Ferre's voluminous flair: silk blouse with huge organza collar and hat by Marina Killery. Modelled by the 'unutterably glamorous' Linda Evangelista, 1991.**

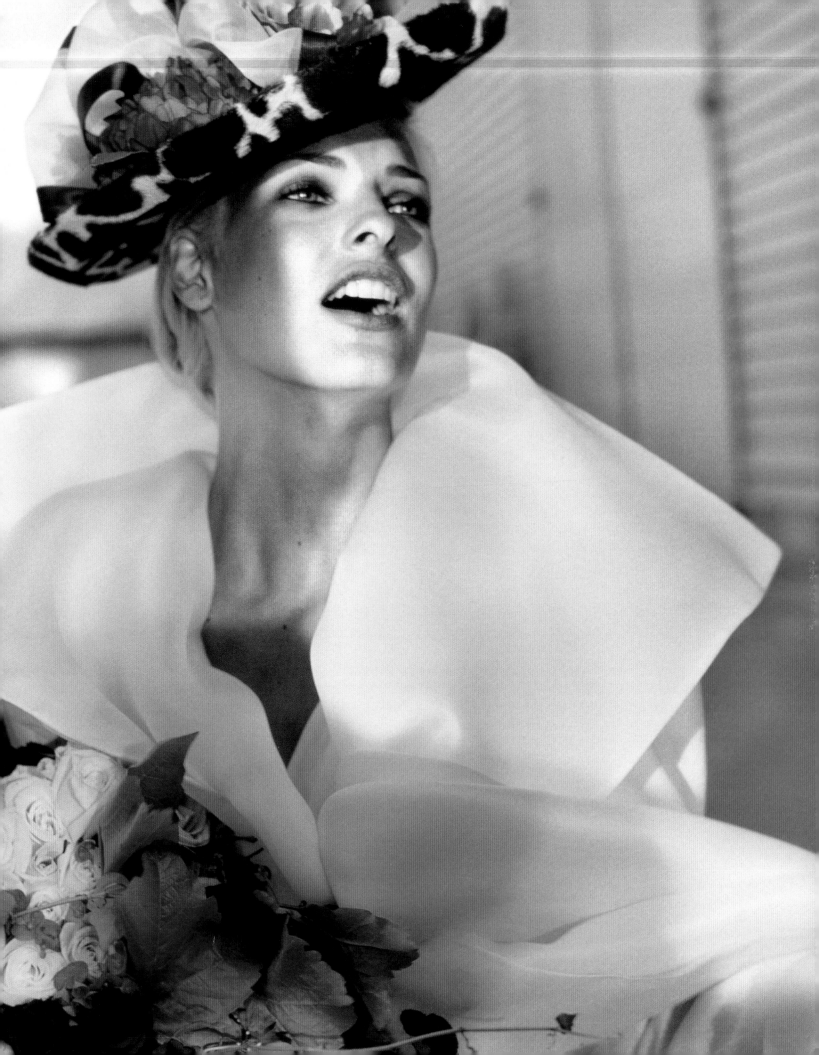

FERRETTI, Alberta

BORN: RICCIONE, ITALY, 1950

That rarest of breeds – clever designer and top flight manufacturer – Alberta Ferretti is one of the most powerful women in Italian fashion. Owner of Aeffe, a high-tech computerized manufacturing complex near Rimini, Ferretti trained at her mother's small atelier before opening her first shop in Cattolica at 18 years old, selling Armani, Krizia and Versace. She switched from selling to designing, and today heads one of the most technologically advanced factories, which has produced collections for Franco Moschino, Rifat Ozbek, Narciso Rodriguez and Jean Paul Gaultier, while producing her own name lines. 'One of my principles is there's no such thing as "It's impossible"', she told *Vogue* in 1992, 'I always try.'

FIORUCCI, Elio

FOUNDED BY ELIO FIORUCCI IN 1962
BORN: MILAN, ITALY, 1935

In the same way that Biba made black lipstick beautiful, Fiorucci made the 1950s fashionable. An inspired retailer, after inheriting his father's footwear business, Elio Fiorucci started to stock hip 1960s' designers (the British contingent included Ossie Clark). Fiorucci was aimed specifically at the youth market, taking inspiration from the 1950s' plastic shoes, bags and jeans – a reversal of roles: American classics with Italian marketing. Colourful and airbrushed, the advertising had a Vargas-Girl slant, with glamorous starlets featured on posters. Fiorucci claims that it was the first company in Italy to show bare breasts in an advertising campaign. Italy went berserk at one particular circular car sticker they produced. 'Fiorucci is fashion. Fiorucci is flash. Fiorucci stores are the best free show in town,' said *The Fiorucci Book* (1981), 'but the difference is all that sex and irony.'

FLETT, John

BORN: CRAWLEY, ENGLAND, 1963
DIED: FLORENCE, ITALY, 1991

John Flett began his career as the star of his year at Central Saint Martins College of Art and Design in London, from where he graduated in 1985. Like John Galliano, Flett had a talent for

unconventional cutting. His first collection caught *Vogue*'s attention and was bought by Joseph and Bloomingdales; he added menswear and diffusion lines to his repertoire in 1986.

In 1989 Flett moved to Paris, working with Claude Montana on his first couture collection for Lanvin. When that didn't work out, he was employed by designer Enrico Coveri in Florence. He was on the verge of signing another deal with the Italian fashion house Zuccoli, when he died tragically young, never fulfilling his early promise like his friend, John Galliano.

FLYTE OSTELL

FOUNDED BY ELLIS FLYTE AND RICHARD OSTELL IN 1991

Both Ellis Flyte and Richard Ostell had survived fashion's school of hard knocks – bankruptcy, backers and being flavour of the month – before joining forces in 1991. Ostell is a superb minimalist designer and Flyte has a flair for theatrical designs; together, they were regarded as the English equivalent to Zoran. Ostell had worked with Romeo Gigli; Flyte in theatre, costume and television.

The Flyte Ostell look – drawstring trousers, fluid tunics, silks and satins – was lauded by the pundits but relentlessly plagiarized. The business folded and they now work separately as consultant designers. As they commented at the time, 'It seems to be what people want. The cut is right, the design is right, the time is right.'

FOALE & TUFFIN

FOUNDED BY MARION FOALE AND SALLY TUFFIN IN 1961

Pioneers of the 1960s, Marion Foale and Sally Tuffin – both graduates of the Royal College of Art in London – started their business from a bedsit in London's Gloucester Road. In 1963 their cottage industry moved to Carnaby Street, which at the time was dotted with haberdasheries and dry-cleaners. Their customers included Jane Asher, Julie Christie and Cilla Black. Foale & Tuffin toured America together with Mary Quant and a contingent of go-go girls. Their first *Vogue* coverage came via an article by Lady Rendlesham.

In 1971 the Piscean partnership reached its natural conclusion and the two designers went their own way professionally. Since 1981 Marion Foale hand-knits in her thatched cottage in the Warwickshire countryside and sells to Barneys New York, Bergdorf Goodman and Harrods. Her ex-partner and long-standing friend, Sally Tuffin, designs ceramics for Dennis China Works in Somerset.

FORD, Tom

Born: Austin, Texas, USA, 1962

The Texan with the Midas touch, Tom Ford has done what every financier dreams about: taken an established label and made it relevant for a new generation. The Gucci phenomenon is the success story that has swept both the fashion industry and the stock market off its feet. Through the canny creation of seasonal must-have icons – in addition to sexy, sophisticated advertising – Ford gives us a perfect example of fashion items which foster huge public demand, and then burn out in time for the next 'big thing'.

Tom Ford moved to Santa Fe, New Mexico, when he was 13 years old. He initially aspired to be an actor and spent six years in Los Angeles. In the late 1970s he arrived in New York, where he frequented the infamous nightclub Studio 54 and studied interior design at Parson's School of Design. He decided to concentrate on fashion instead and ended up as a senior designer at Cathy Hardwick's studio on Seventh Avenue. Two years later Ford had moved to Perry Ellis as design director of Women's America Division. In 1990 he relocated again – this time to Milan, where he worked for Dawn Mello at Gucci, eventually taking over from her when she moved back to New York in 1994 to head up department store, Bergdorf Goodman.

In 1992 Ford designed his first menswear collection. The tide turned in his favour in March 1995. Celebrity backing and advertising campaigns, photographed by Mario Testino, followed. Famous for photographing the world's most beautiful women, Testino presented Ford's overtly sexy designs in a dramatic, deeply glamorous, light.

Ford's fashion inspiration came from his grandmother: 'She was an Auntie Mame character,' Ford told American *Vogue* in 1999, 'with six husbands and a closet full of Courrèges pantsuits, coral bangles and I Dream of Jeannie falls.' Still harbouring a secret desire to tread the boards, Ford has a Hollywood agent who vets scripts for him. Ford works on instinct. In 1999, when Gucci was under threat from a takeover, Ford made a multi-million dollar decision for a new investor over lunch. 'What can I say?' he told *Vanity Fair* later, 'I'm a Virgo.'

RIGHT **Taking Gucci to its natural conclusion, Tom Ford designs the ultimate funnel neck coat for winter 1999, tied at the waist with a leather thong.**

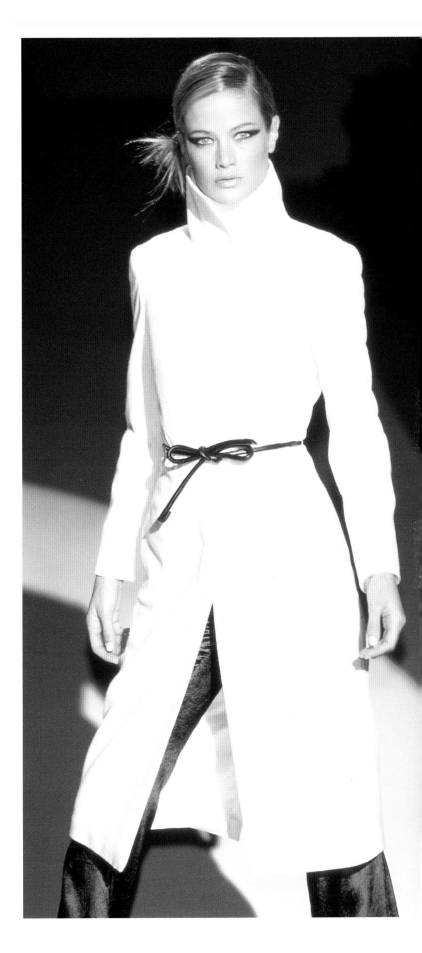

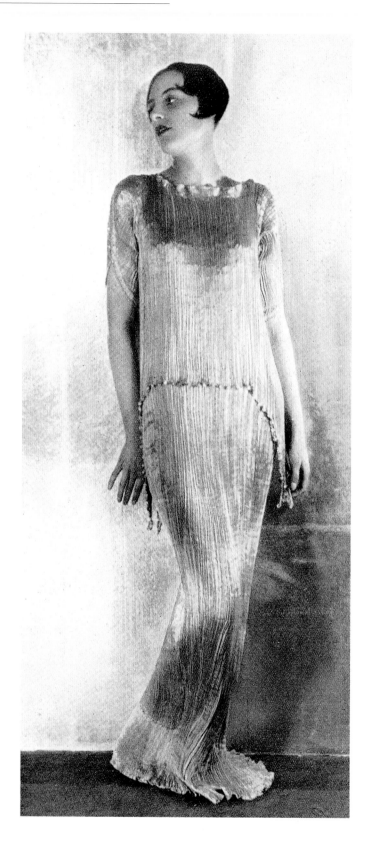

FORTUNY, Mariano

BORN: GRANADA, SPAIN, 1871
DIED: VENICE, ITALY, 1949

Mariano Fortuny was a visionary, Renaissance man and creator of revolutionary fabrics. His Delphos gown, devised in 1907 and patented two years later, was a masterpiece of fabric and form: a free-flowing revelation in a period of restriction, made from a tube of pleated silk. In one stroke of genius, Fortuny embodied the principles of the aesthetic and rational dress movements, whose supporters relentlessly campaigned for the abolition of torturous corsetry. His dresses were drawn on Greek lines, suspended from the shoulder and later decorated with Venetian glass beads. 'This invention is related to a type of garment derived from the Classical robe,' stated Fortuny's original patent description, 'but its design is so shaped and arranged that it can be worn and adjusted with ease and comfort.'

Son of a distinguished Spanish painter, Fortuny came to Venice when his mother, Cecilia de Madrazo, moved to the seventeenth-century Palazzo Martinengo after his father's death. Fortuny was a natural-born textile designer, producing Knossos printed scarves from 1906, opening a showroom for the sale of textiles and clothing in Venice and establishing his own factory for printing fabrics in 1919. Fortuny's talents were not limited to his most famous invention: he developed techniques of printing and over-painting on velvets and cottons, photographed stunning panoramic views of Venice and even invented a new kind of photographic paper. In all, he was an incredible sculptor, artist, stage designer, scientist and chemist – refining and reinventing everything he touched, from theatrical sets to lighting.

The most sensitive colourist of the twentieth century, Fortuny often dipped lengths of silk several times to achieve the precise tone. His perfectionism knew no bounds. Together with the standard Delphos design, Fortuny also patented his pleating methods: the intricacies remain a mystery, but in layman's terms this involved a complicated and arduous process of running the irregular, horizontal folds of silk between copper plates and ceramic tubes.

The Fortuny Museum, in the Palazzo Pesaro, Venice, stands as a monument to Italy's most notable fashion genius. Timeless and modern in the truest sense of the word, Fortuny designs were featured in *Vogue* in 1927 and again almost 50 years on – its advocates spanned half a century, from Isadora Duncan to Julie Christie. Unlike most wearable antiques, original Fortuny's have not disintegrated with time. Still mesmerizing and stunning in the flesh, Fortuny gowns are worn, collected and lusted after – an amazing feat after almost a century in circulation.

ABOVE **Fortuny's masterpiece of 1927: a tea gown in perpendicular, finely pleated satin, with opalescent beads on the hem.**

OPPOSITE **Julie Christie in Venice, wearing a Fortuny gown borrowed from ardent collector and artist, Mrs Liselotte Hohs Manera, 1973.**

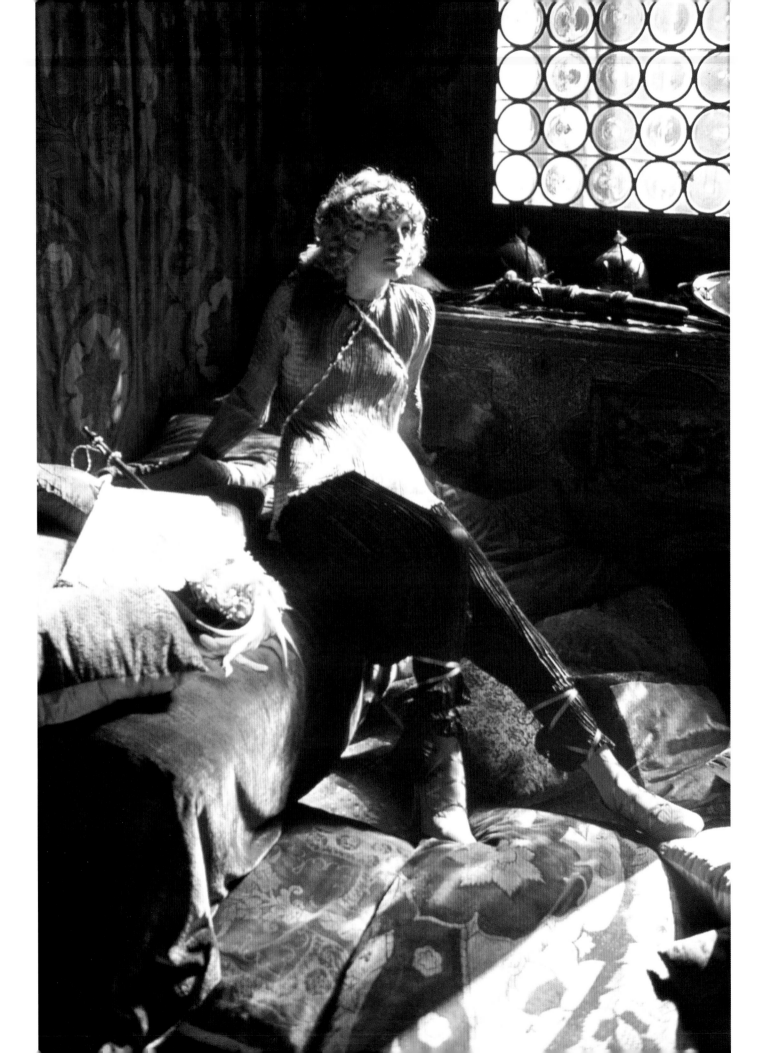

FOX, Frederick

BORN: URANA, AUSTRALIA, 1931

Frederick Fox, England's most distinguished milliner, is an Australian who spent his childhood on a farm in New South Wales. During the Second World War, he created new hats by cutting up old ones and reconstructing them. At 17 years old he moved to Sydney, where he visited other milliners – first Henriette Lamotte, who pointed him in the direction of a Mrs Normoyle. Nine months later he moved to Phyl Clarkson, where he stayed for ten years. He travelled to London via Paris and secured a job with Otto Lucas. It was, by his own admission, a tough learning curve: 'I was 26, looked 15 and was in charge of a table of 40 women old enough to be my mother.' He moved on to Mitzi Lorenz, then to Langée in Brook Street, London, which he took over in 1964, and then moved to his present premises in Bond Street.

Fox began making hats to complement the Queen's wardrobe, designed by Hardy Amies, in 1968. His first five hats were for a tour of Chile and Argentina. He received his royal warrant in 1974 as Milliner to HM The Queen and was awarded an LVO in the Queen's 1999 birthday honours list. At one time he hatted eight royal ladies – including Queen Elizabeth the Queen Mother, Princess Alice and Diana, Princess of Wales.

Fox's talent is not limited to creating hats for Ascot, chic weddings and royal tours. He has worked with Red or Dead, and designed the white leather crash helmets that appeared in Stanley Kubrik's classic film *2001, A Space Odyssey* (1968).

FRATINI, Gina

BORN: KOBE, JAPAN, 1934

One of the key instigators of the 1960s romantic movement, Gina Fratini had Irish parentage but was raised in Japan. Her father, the Honourable Somerset Butler, was twin brother of the Earl of Carrick. In 1947 Fratini attended the Royal College of Art in London and then joined the Katherine Dunham dance group, assisting the costume and set designer, John Platt. She also designed clothes independently, and continued to produce private commissions after she married jazz guitarist David Goldberg in 1954.

In 1965, on marrying Renato Fratini, she established her own business, which continued successfully until 1989. Before Marc Bohan joined Hartnell in 1990, Gina Fratini was a guest designer there: 'It was the first time I could just create without thinking of the business. It was wonderful. What a treat and a joy it was just to design.'

FREUD, Bella

BORN: LONDON, ENGLAND, 1961

Bella Freud – daughter of artist Lucien and sister of novelist Esther – designs clothes like those she wears: schoolgirl coats and lean shapes. Her logo, drawn by her father Lucien, depicts his whippet, Pluto.

Freud worked as an assistant in Vivienne Westwood's Seditionaries shop in London's King's Road before going to Rome to study design at the Accademia di Costuma di Moda. On her return in 1984 she worked with Westwood on the 'Mini-Crini' collection and became her assistant until she set up her own collection of 30 pieces in 1989. Her first show was in 1993.

Bella Freud had a bohemian childhood, and the year spent in Morocco with her mother and sister was immortalized in Esther's novel, *Hideous Kinky* (1992). She has been captured on canvas many times. Freud's father – who critics regard as the greatest living artist – often slips into the shows unnoticed.

OPPOSITE **Bella Freud's 'weird, wonderful, mismatched colours': canary wool twill jacket, Neapolitan merino wool leggings and leather platforms, 1992.**

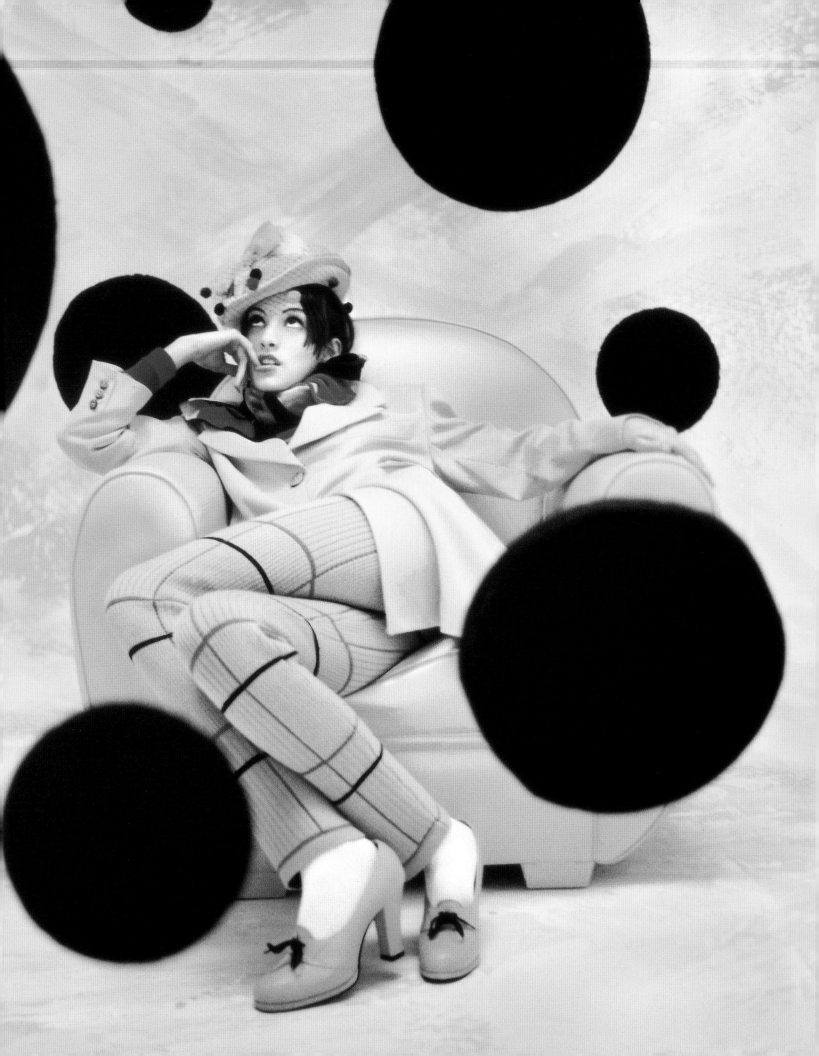

INDEX

PICTURE CREDITS

The publishers would like to thank the following sources for their kind permission to reproduce the pictures in this book:

t: top, b: bottom, l: left, r: right, tl: top left, tr: top right, bl: bottom left, br: bottom right, bc: bottom centre, bcl: bottom centre left, bcr: bottom centre right.

All images © *Vogue*, The Condé Nast Publications Ltd.

B.D.V/Corbis (jacket)
Eric Boman 16,
Rene Bouche 30
Pierre Cardin 25
Oleg Cassini 26
Castaldi 57
Alex Chatelain 17, 21, 48, 50,
Willie Christie 4, 15,
Henry Clarke 13, 43,
Clifford Coffin 44
Patrick Demarchelier 1, 7,
Arthur Elgort 9,
Perry Ellis 49,
Lee Creelman Erickson 11,
Hans Feurer 10,
Mikael Jansson 28,
Neil Kirk 40
Kelly Klein 23,
Kim Knott 42
Peter Lindbergh 46
Frances McLaughlin-Gill 12,
Herbert Matter 52
Raymond Meier 20,
Steven Meisel 3, 36,
David Montgomery 32, 33, 34
Tom Munro 33,

Helmut Newton 27,
Norman Parkinson 8
David Sims 37,
Mario Testino 31, 45
Javier Vallhonrat 53, 59
Justin de Villeneuve 18, 19
Albert Watson 22

Every effort has been made to acknowledge correctly and contact the source and/copyright holder of each picture, and Carlton Books Limited apologizes for any unintentional errors or omissions which will be corrected in future editions of this book.

ACKNOWLEDGEMENTS

Very special thanks to Erika Frei for her encouragement
and advice on the fine art of tact and diplomacy.
To Joyce Douglas for being there.

Thank you to Vogue's superb library staff
– Darlene Maxwell, Chris Pipe, Nancy Kim, headed by
the brilliant Lisa Hodgkins – for their support, good humour
and company throughout this project.

Two people who were fundamental: endless thanks
to Francesca Harrison, picture editor, for being calm,
efficient and having a lovely eye. Emily Wheeler-Bennett,
Condé Nast's editorial business and rights director,
for being a complete professional and friend.

This book is dedicated to my mother, father and
brother Billy with love.